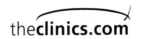

FOOT AND ANKLE CLINICS

Arthroscopy and Endoscopy of the Foot and Ankle

GUEST EDITOR
C. Niek van Dijk, MD, PhD

CONSULTING EDITOR
Mark S. Myerson, MD

June 2006 • Volume 11 • Number 2

SAUNDERS

An Imprint of Elsevier, Inc.
PHILADELPHIA   LONDON   TORONTO   MONTREAL   SYDNEY   TOKYO

W.B. SAUNDERS COMPANY
A Division of Elsevier Inc.

1600 John F. Kennedy Blvd., Suite 1800, Philadelphia, PA 19103-2899

http://www.theclinics.com

FOOT AND ANKLE CLINICS
June 2006
Editor: Debora Dellapena

Volume 11, Number 2
ISSN 1083-7515
ISBN 1-4160-3505-2

Foot and Ankle Clinics (ISSN 1083-7515) is published quarterly by W.B. Saunders, 360 Park Avenue South, New York, NY 10010-1710. Months of publication are March, June, September, and December. Business and Editorial Offices: 1600 John F. Kennedy Blvd., Suite 1800, Philadelphia, PA 19103-2899. Accounting and Circulation Offices: 6277 Sea Harbor Drive, Orlando, FL 32887-4800. Periodicals postage paid at New York, NY, and additional mailing offices. Subscription prices are $170.00 per year for US individuals, $245.00 per year for US institutions, $85.00 per year for US students and residents, $190.00 per year for Canadian individuals, $285.00 per year for Canadian institutions, $230.00 for international individuals, $285.00 for international institutions and $110.00 per year for Canadian and foreign students residents. To receive student/resident rate, orders must be accompanied by name of affiliated institution, date of term, and the *signature* of program/residency coordinator on institution letterhead. Orders will be billed at individual rate until proof of status is received. Foreign air speed delivery is included in all *Clinics* subscription prices. All prices are subject to change without notice. POSTMASTER: Send address changes to *Foot and Ankle Clinics*, Elsevier Periodicals Customer Service, 6277 Harbor Drive, Orlando, FL 32887-4800. **Customer Service: 1-800-654-2452 (US). From outside of the US, call 1-407-345-1000.**

Printed in the United States of America.

CONSULTING EDITOR

MARK S. MYERSON, MD, President, American Orthopaedic Foot and Ankle Society; Director, The Institute for Foot and Ankle Reconstruction, Mercy Medical Center, Baltimore, Maryland

GUEST EDITOR

C. NIEK VAN DIJK, MD, PhD, Professor and Head, Department of Orthopaedic Surgery University Hospital, Academic Medical Center, Amsterdam, The Netherlands

CONTRIBUTORS

LIJKELE BEIMERS, MD, Department of Orthopaedic Surgery University Hospital, Academic Medical Center, Amsterdam, The Netherlands

GYTHE H. BULSTRA, MD, Department of Orthopaedic Surgery, Academic Medical Center, Amsterdam, The Netherlands

JASPER DE VRIES, MD, Research Fellow, Department of Orthopaedic Surgery, Academic Medical Center, Amsterdam, The Netherlands

RYAN M. DOPIRAK, MD, Sports Medicine Fellow, Southern California Orthopedic Institute, Van Nuys, California

RICHARD D. FERKEL, MD, Director of Sports Medicine Fellowship, Attending Surgeon, Southern California Orthopedic Institute, Van Nuys, California

CAROL FREY, MD, Fellowship Director, West Coast Sports Medicine; Assistant Clinical Professor, Department of Orthopaedic Surgery, University of California Los Angeles, Manhattan Beach, California

PAU GOLANÓ, MD, Laboratory of Arthroscopic and Surgical Anatomy, Department of Pathology and Experimental Therapeutics, Human Anatomy Unit, University of Barcelona, Barcelona, Spain

VÍCTOR GÖTZENS, MD, PhD, Laboratory of Arthroscopic and Surgical Anatomy, Department of Pathology and Experimental Therapeutics (Human Anatomy Unit), University of Barcelona, Barcelona, Spain

LÁSZLÓ HANGODY, MD, PhD, DSc, Uzsoki Hospital, Department of Orthopaedics, Budapest, Hungary

ROVER KRIPS, MD, PhD, Resident Orthopaedic Surgery, Department of Orthopaedic Surgery, Academic Medical Center, Amsterdam, The Netherlands

PAUL G.M. OLSTHOORN, MD, Orthopedic Surgeon, Slotervaart Hospital, Amsterdam, The Netherlands

LUIS PÉREZ-CARRO, MD, PhD, Department of Orthopedic and Trauma Surgery, Centro Médico Lealtad, Santander, Spain

PETER E. SCHOLTEN, MD, Department of Orthopaedic Surgery, Kliniek Klein Rosendael, Rozendaal, The Netherlands

FERRY STEENSTRA, MD, Orthopaedic Surgeon in Training, Academic Medical Center Amsterdam, Utrecht, The Netherlands

JAMES W. STONE, MD, Assistant Clinical Professor of Orthopedic Surgery, Medical College of Wisconsin, Milwaukee, Wisconsin

IMRE SZERB, MD, PhD, Uzsoki Hospital, Department of Orthopaedics, Budapest, Hungary

JOHANNES L. TOL, MD, PhD, Department of Sports Medicine, Medical Center Haaglanden, Leidschendam, The Netherlands

C. NIEK VAN DIJK, MD, PhD, Professor and Head, Department of Orthopaedic Surgery University Hospital, Academic Medical Center, Amsterdam, The Netherlands

JORDI VEGA, MD, Department of Orthopedic and Trauma Surgery, "La Mútua," Granollers, Barcelona, Spain; Laboratory of Arthroscopic and Surgical Anatomy, Department of Pathology and Experimental Therapeutics (Human Anatomy Unit), University of Barcelona, Barcelona, Spain

MAARTJE ZENGERINK, MD, Department of Orthopaedic Surgery, Academic Medical Center, University of Amsterdam, Amsterdam, The Netherlands

CONTRIBUTORS

CONTENTS

with particular emphasis on specific anatomic details that are often omitted or little known and that have considerable clinical interest because of their involvement in soft tissue syndrome.

The anterior ankle impingement syndrome is a clinical pain syndrome that is characterized by anterior ankle pain on (hyper) dorsiflexion. The plain radiographs often are negative in patients who have anteromedial impingement. An oblique view is recommended in these patients. Arthroscopic excision of soft tissue overgrowths and osteophytes is an effective way of treating anterior impingement of the ankle in patients who have no narrowing of the joint space. For grade II lesions (osteophytes secondary to arthritis with joint space narrowing) arthroscopic treatment is a good option, because no other therapeutic option is available with the exception of an arthrodesis or prothesis.

The ankle joint is the most congruent joint of the human body. Stability is provided by the bony configuration of the ankle mortise and the talar dome and by the ankle ligaments. During ankle motions, rotation and translation around and along the movement axes occur. Soft tissue stability is provided mainly by the ligaments. This article discusses ankle instability, injuries, and reconstruction.

Osteochondral ankle defects cause various symptoms including pain, swelling, and limited range of motion. When surgical treatment is necessary, several treatment options exist. Arthroscopic debridement and drilling, arthroscopic autologous osteochondral transplantation (mosaiclasty), and autologous chondrocyte transplantation are discussed more extensively. Treatment results of each technique are discussed, and a guideline for treatment is presented.

Surgical options are limited for the patient who has symptomatic severe ankle joint degeneration that is unresponsive to nonoperative treatment. Arthrodesis of the tibiotalar joint is a procedure that can produce a pain-free ankle that can withstand the rigors of daily life, even in a young, high-demand, working individual. Minimally invasive orthopedic techniques have been applied to ankle arthrodesis, and arthroscopic ankle fusion has been shown to be an effective technique to achieve tibiotalar arthrodesis, with high rates of fusion and low rates of complication. This article covers indications, contraindications, and procedural techniques for arthroscopic ankle arthrodesis. Results of arthroscopic versus open ankle arthrodesis are compared.

The subtalar joint is a complex and functionally important joint of the lower extremity. It plays a major role in the movement of inversion and eversion of the foot. With the development of small-joint arthroscopes and instrumentation, surgeons became interested in posterior subtalar joint arthroscopy. Diagnostic and therapeutic indications for this technique have increased; however, arthroscopic subtalar surgery is technically difficult and should be performed by an experienced arthroscopist. The number of reports dealing with posterior subtalar arthroscopy remains relatively small.

Hindfoot pain can be caused by a variety of pathologies; most of these can be diagnosed and treated by means of endoscopy. The main indications are posterior tibial tenosynovectomy, diagnosis of a peroneus brevis length rupture, peroneal tendon athesiolysis, flexor hallucis longus release, os trigonum removal, endoscopic treatment for retrocalcaneal bursitis, endoscopic treatment for achilles (peri)tendinopathy, and treatment of ankle joint or subtalar joint pathology. The advantages of endoscopic hindfoot surgery over open surgery are less morbidity, reduction of postoperative pain, outpatient treatment, and functional postoperative treatment. This two-portal hindfoot endoscopy approach is a safe, reliable, and exciting method to diagnose and treat a variety of posterior ankle problems and offers a good alternative to open surgery.

Tendoscopy of the peroneal tendons is a useful tool to diagnose and treat peroneal tendon disorders. Endoscopic ankle surgery is followed by a functional postoperative treatment and offers the advantages of less morbidity, reduction of postoperative pain, and outpatient surgery. The article describes the technique and results of peroneal tendoscopy performed in 23 patients between 1995 and 2000.

FORTHCOMING ISSUES

September 2006
Instability and Impingement Syndrome
Nicola Maffulli, MD, MS, PhD, FRCS(Orth), *Guest Editor*

December 2006
The Diabetic Foot and Ankle
Brian G. Donley, MD, *Guest Editor*

March 2007
Complex Salvage of Ankle and Hindfoot Deformity
Donald R. Bohay, MD, and
John G. Anderson, MD, *Guest Editors*

RECENT ISSUES

March 2006
Posttraumatic Reconstruction of the Foot and Ankle
Alastair S.E. Younger, MB ChB, MSc, ChM, FRCSC,
Guest Editor

December 2005
Orthobiologics
Sheldon S. Lin, MD, *Guest Editor*

September 2005
The Calcaneus
Paul J. Juliano, MD, *Guest Editor*

THE CLINICS ARE NOW AVAILABLE ONLINE!

http://www.theclinics.com

ELSEVIER
SAUNDERS

Foot Ankle Clin N Am
11 (2006) xi–xii

FOOT AND
ANKLE CLINICS

Preface

Arthroscopy and Endoscopy of the Foot and Ankle

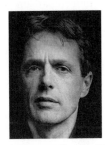

C. Niek van Dijk, MD, PhD
Guest Editor

Significant progress has been made in the field of endoscopic foot and ankle surgery over the last 25 years. Arthroscopy of the ankle joint has become an important diagnostic and therapeutic procedure for the detection and treatment of chronic and posttraumatic problems. Additional radiographs, such as the anteromedial impingement view, the heel rise view, or the posterior impingement view, are important for the confirmation of a clinical diagnosis and for planning a treatment.

Anterior ankle problems include soft tissue and bony impingement, synovitis, loose bodies, and ossicles. Complaints located more centrally can originate from an osteochondral defect or from arthrosis. For preoperative planning, CT scanning offers better information than MR imaging. Therapy is guided mainly by the size of the lesion. For primary lesions, the best option for treatment is currently debridement and bone marrow stimulation. Large cystic lesions can be treated by retrograde drilling and bone grafting. Secondary lesions can be treated by osteochondral transplants or chondrocyte grafts.

Because of their nature and their deep location, posterior ankle problems pose a diagnostic and therapeutic challenge. By means of a two-portal hindfoot approach, with the patient in the prone position, posterior ankle joint problems such as loose bodies, ossicles, osteophytes, or osteochondral defects can be treated. In a case of a posterior ankle impingement syndrome, bony impediments

1083-7515/06/$ – see front matter © 2006 Elsevier Inc. All rights reserved.
doi:10.1016/j.fcl.2006.04.001

like an os trigonum can be detached and removed. This approach offers access to the deep portion of the deltoid ligament, the posterior syndesmotic ligament, the posterior talofibular ligament, and the flexor hallucis longus tendon, as well as the posterior compartment of the subtalar joint. Pathology of these structures can be detected and treated.

Tendoscopy of the peroneal tendons, the posterior tibial tendon, and the achilles tendon offers access to these tendons for diagnostic and therapeutic purposes. For chronic retrocalcaneal bursitis, endoscopical calcaneoplasty has been demonstrated to show several advantages, including low morbidity, functional after-treatment, outpatient treatment, excellent scar healing, a short recovery time, and quicker sport resumption, in comparison to open techniques. The same advantages apply to most of the endoscopic techniques described in this issue. Having read this issue of the *Foot and Ankle Clinics*, I expect surgeons familiar with the arthroscope, as well as their patients, to find these arthroscopic techniques a more rewarding experience.

C. Niek van Dijk, MD, PhD
Department of Orthopaedic Surgery
Academic Medical Center
P.O. Box 22700
1100 DD Amsterdam, The Netherlands
E-mail address: c.n.vandijk@amc.uva.nl

ELSEVIER
SAUNDERS

Foot Ankle Clin N Am
11 (2006) 253–273

FOOT AND
ANKLE CLINICS

Ankle Anatomy for the Arthroscopist. Part I: The Portals

Pau Golanó, MD[a,*], Jordi Vega, MD[a,b],
Luis Pérez-Carro, MD, PhD[c], Víctor Götzens, MD, PhD[a]

[a]Laboratory of Arthroscopic and Surgical Anatomy, Department of Pathology and
Experimental Therapeutics (Human Anatomy Unit), University of Barcelona,
c/ Feixa Llarga s/n (Campus Bellvitge), L'Hospitalet de Llobregat, Barcelona 08907, Spain
[b]Department of Orthopedic and Trauma Surgery, "La Mútua," Granollers, Barcelona, Spain
[c]Department of Orthopedic and Trauma Surgery, Centro Médico Lealtad, Santander, Spain

Over the last decade, arthroscopy of the ankle has become an important tool for the diagnosis and treatment of numerous pathologies. The considerable increase in the use of endoscopic techniques has led to significant changes in the field of orthopedic surgery and a new concept of human anatomy. The typical visualization in three dimensions on the part of surgeons and anatomists has become a two-dimensional, magnified view with the capability to observe anatomic structures that cannot be accessed by open surgery or dissection without altering their location or morphology. Because endoscopic procedures are performed using small incisions through which instruments are passed from the surface to the depths of the area under treatment, an anatomic focus is required that is based on the relationships between the structures susceptible to lesion and the arthroscopic access routes or portals.

Hence, adequate knowledge of the anatomy of the joint to be treated should cover not only the most common anatomic configurations (extra-articular and intra-articular) in statistical terms but also the possible anatomic variations to avoid confusion and serious technical errors. This anatomic knowledge is particularly important in arthroscopy of the ankle because of the significant risk of associated complications, which can be prevented or decreased only by profound familiarity with the anatomy of the region and the use of a "protocolled," reproducible technique [1].

---

* Corresponding author.
E-mail address: pgolano@ub.edu (P. Golanó).

Some of the most important aspects of arthroscopic procedures that have an anatomic basis as their focus are (1) the use of incisions that only affect the skin and are placed parallel to the neighboring tendinous and vasculonervous structures, which run from the leg to the foot in a proximal to distal direction; (2) the use of blunt dissection with a vascular or mosquito clamp until the joint capsule is reached; (3) the use of blunt trocars to avoid injury to the articular cartilage (a frequent problem, particularly in arthroscopists who have limited experience); (4) the use of arthroscopy sheaths with no lateral window to avoid leakage of irrigation fluid into surrounding tissues and that are interchangeable to prevent soft tissue trauma by repetitive insertion of the instruments; and (5) the use of arthroscopic cannulas to introduce motorized instruments [2,3].

In 1931, Burman [4], a pioneer in establishing the anatomic basis of arthroscopy of the ankle and foot, stated that the ankle joint "is not suitable for arthroscopy." He maintained that the joint space was extremely narrow and traction could not separate the articular surfaces. Although he believed access to

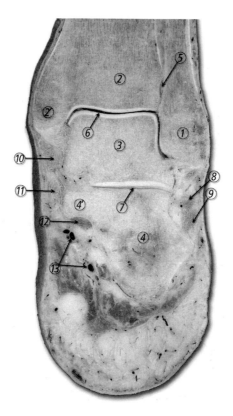

Fig. 1. Frontal section of the ankle joint. 1, lateral malleolus; 2, tibia; 2', medial malleolus; 3, talus; 4, calcaneus; 4', sustentaculum tali; 5, tibiofibular syndesmosis; 6, talocrural joint; 7, posterior subtalar joint; 8, peroneus brevis tendon; 9, peroneus longus tendon; 10, tibialis posterior tendon; 11, flexor digitorum longus tendon; 12, flexor hallucis longus tendon; 13, lateral and medial plantar artery.

the posterior region was not feasible, he described the possibility of accessing the joint through an anterior approach located lateral to the extensor tendons and concluded that perhaps "something" could be done in a live patient with a smaller arthroscope. Effectively, the technologic advances that have taken place since that time and particularly in the last decades have yielded smaller-diameter arthroscopes than those used by Burman and systems of traction/distraction that allow better access to the joint, thereby increasing the indications for the technique.

The advantages of arthroscopy for treating the ankle and foot are similar to those observed in other joints; however, the fast increase in the popularity of this technique is also due to the fact that other noninvasive methods are not suitable for the diagnosis of certain ankle alterations. This is particularly true for the soft tissue lesions known as "soft tissue impingement syndrome," which together with osteochondral lesions are among the main indications for arthroscopy [5].

The authors' objective in this article is to present the anatomy of the ankle joint specifically from the perspective of arthroscopy, omitting general and other considerations that are not highly relevant in arthroscopic practice.

The ankle joint or talocrural articulation is formed by the articular surfaces of the distal tibial and fibular epiphyses and the talus in its superior, lateral, and medial aspects. The morphology of these surfaces forms a hinge-type synovial joint with a single axis of movement (bimalleolar axis) that allows dorsiflexion (flexion) and plantar flexion (extension) of the ankle and foot in the sagittal plane. Because of this configuration and the fact that the ankle is a load-bearing joint, the interarticular space is narrow, making insertion of arthroscopic instruments between the articular surfaces difficult (Fig. 1). Hence, articular distraction systems are required to perform complete arthroscopic inspection of the joint.

Landmarks

The anatomic landmarks of bone and tissue in the ankle joint are easily palpated and should be delimited on the patient's skin with a dermographic marker. Landmarks are essential for proper positioning of the portals and facilitate orientation during the procedure despite the edema associated with the technique. The following landmarks are the most important: (1) both malleoli (lateral and medial); (2) the anterior joint line, which is easily palpated by moving the joint in dorsiflexion–plantar flexion and located approximately 2 cm proximal to the tip of the lateral malleolus and 1 cm proximal to the tip of the medial malleolus; (3) the tibialis anterior tendon, fibularis tertius tendon, and calcaneal or Achilles tendon; (4) vascular landmarks such as the great saphenous vein, which runs in front of the medial malleolus, and the superficial peroneal nerve with its dividing branches: the medial and intermedial dorsal cutaneous nerves. These vessels are easily identified in thin patients when inversion of the foot is performed. Neural structures such as the sural nerve, which usually runs 2 cm

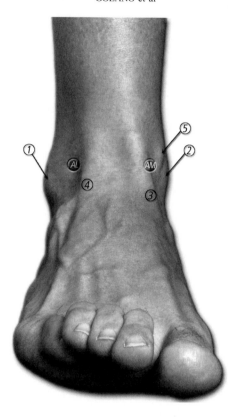

Fig. 2. Cutaneous landmarks of anterior view of the ankle. AL, anterolateral portal; AM, anteromedial portal; 1, lateral malleolus; 2, medial malleolus; 3, tibialis anterior tendon; 4, extensor digitorum longus tendon; 5, great saphenous vein.

posterior and distal to the lateral malleolus, together with the small saphenous vein, are also easily palpated (Figs. 2 and 3) [2].

Arthroscopic portals

The numerous arthroscopic portals described for the ankle can be grouped into anterior, posterior, transmalleolar, and transtalar. The use of some of these portals involves considerable technical difficulty or an elevated potential for neurovascular lesion, and for these reasons, they have fallen into disuse.

The first description of the anteromedial, anterolateral, and posterior portals of the ankle was reported by Watanabe in 1972 [6]. In later years, investigators such as Ikehuchi [7], Chen [8], Drez and colleagues [9,10], Parisien and colleagues [11–13], and Andrews [14] described additional portals and the extra-articular

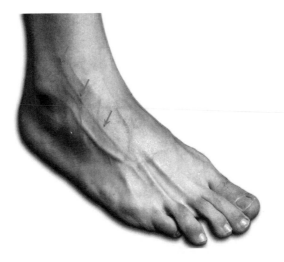

Fig. 3. Subcutaneous course of the superficial peroneal nerve (intermediate dorsal cutaneous branch), indicated with arrows.

and intra-articular anatomy of the ankle and standardized the technique, which was ultimately popularized by Ferkel and Fischer [15]. Subsequently, several investigators described new portals to fill the need to access specific regions of the joint, particularly the central and posterior areas (Box 1) [16–20]. This need also led to the development of various systems of distraction to allow easy, safe, and more complete visualization of the ankle joint [21–29].

Owing to the fact that all the portals run through an anatomic region surrounded by numerous neurovascular structures susceptible to injury, several anatomic studies to assess the potential for lesion to each of them have been published (Fig. 4) [15,16,30–37].

Anterior portals

Anteromedial portal

The anteromedial portal is the first to be performed. It is established just medial to the tibialis anterior tendon at the anterior joint line of the ankle and coinciding with a soft spot, a visible and palpable depression seen when the ankle is in dorsiflexion. There is a potential for injury to the saphenous nerve and the great saphenous vein, which at this level, divides into numerous branches that communicate with the deep venous system (see Fig. 4; Figs. 5 and 6). These structures lie at a mean safe distance of 9 mm (3–16 mm) for the saphenous vein and 7.4 mm (0–17 mm) for the saphenous nerve [30]. Although some investigators consider these structures risk-free [32], Chen [8] reported one case of saphenous vein lesion in 67 ankles treated with arthroscopy and Ferkel and col-

---

Box 1. Arthroscopic portals described for the ankle joint

Anterior portals

　　Anteromedial
　　Accessory anteromedial
　　Anterocentral
　　Medial midline portal [18]
　　Anterolateral
　　Accessory anterolateral

Posterior portals

　　Posteromedial
　　Accessory posteromedial
　　Modified posteromedial [17]
　　TransAchilles [16]
　　Posterolateral
　　Accessory posterolateral
　　Coaxial portals [20]
　　Endoscopic portals [19]

Transmalleolar portals

　　Medial
　　Lateral

Transtalar portals

　　Medial
　　Lateral

---

leagues [5] described 27 neurologic complications, 5 corresponding to saphenous nerve injuries.

At the anterior edge of the tibia, where it joins with the medial malleolus, there is a notch (medial notch of Harty) [38] that provides the anteromedial portal with additional space to allow easier passage of the instruments in the anteroposterior direction [39] (Fig. 7).

Anterolateral portal

The anterolateral portal is created at the anterior joint line just lateral to the peroneus tertius tendon (present in 90% of cases) [40] or, in its absence, lateral to

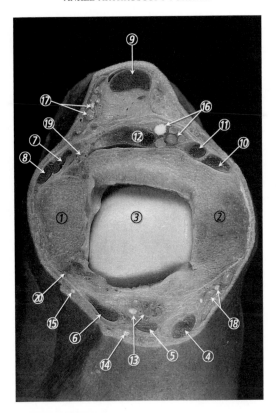

Fig. 4. Transverse section at the level of the ankle joint. 1, lateral malleolus; 2, medial malleolus; 3, talus; 4, tibialis anterior tendon; 5, extensor hallucis longus tendon; 6, extensor digitorum longus and peroneus tertius tendons; 7, peroneus brevis tendon; 8, peroneus longus tendon; 9, calcaneal tendon; 10, tibialis posterior tendon; 11, flexor digitorum longus; 12, flexor hallucis tendon (musculotendinous); 13, deep peroneal nerve and anterior tibial artery and veins; 14, medial dorsal cutaneous nerve (medial terminal branch of superficial peroneal nerve); 15, intermediate dorsal cutaneous nerve (lateral terminal branch of superficial peroneal nerve); 16, posterior tibial nerve and posterior tibial artery and veins; 17, sural nerve and small saphenous vein; 18, saphenous nerve and great saphenous vein; 19, posterior peroneal artery; 20, anterior peroneal artery.

the extensor digitorum longus tendons. The main structure at risk of injury when performing this portal is the intermediate dorsal cutaneous nerve (the lateral branch of the superficial peroneal nerve) [41] (see Figs 4 and 5). Most of the complications described in arthroscopy of the ankle involve this nerve [5,42,43].

The superficial peroneal nerve, which is the motor for the muscles of the lateral compartment of the leg (peroneus longus and peroneus brevis) and the sensory nerve for the greater part of the dorsal foot, has been the subject of numerous anatomic studies [30–33,44–46]. After providing motor innervation, the superficial peroneal nerve runs along the lateral intermuscular septum and penetrates the crural fascia, where it becomes a sensory nerve. The point of

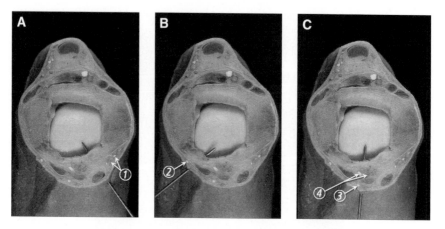

Fig. 5. Transverse section at the level of the ankle joint. (*A*) Anteromedial portal. 1, saphenous nerve and great saphenous vein. (*B*) Anterolateral portal. 2, intermediate dorsal cutaneous nerve (lateral terminal branch of superficial peroneal nerve). (*C*) Anterocentral portal. 3, medial dorsal cutaneous nerve (medial terminal branch of superficial peroneal nerve); 4, deep peroneal nerve and anterior tibial artery and veins.

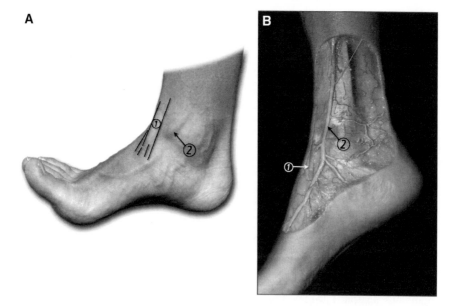

Fig. 6. (*A*) Medial view of the ankle. (*B*) Anatomic dissection (veins are filled with blue latex for better identification). 1, tibialis anterior tendon; 2, great saphenous vein and communicans branches.

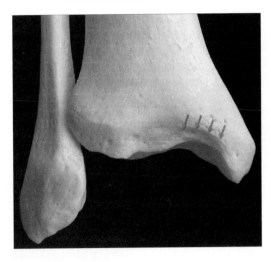

Fig. 7. Anterior view of the distal tibial and peroneal epiphyses. Note the notch of Harty (*arrows*) at the anterior edge of the tibia, where it joins the medial malleolus.

penetration varies, although it is usually found at a distance from the medial malleolus equivalent to one-third the length of the tibia [44]. Distal from this point, the superficial peroneal nerve usually divides into two branches: the more laterally located intermediate dorsal cutaneous nerve and the medial dorsal cutaneous nerve (Fig. 8). Various types or patterns have been described according to the level and manner in which the superficial peroneal nerve divides into its branches [31,32,44–46]. The distance from the intermediate dorsal cutaneous nerve to the anterolateral portal has been quantified [30,31,33]. Feiwell and Frey [30] reported a mean distance of 6.2 mm (0–24 mm). In the authors' experience, these data are not very useful because it is almost impossible to know the patient's nerve distribution. Nevertheless, the arthroscopist should be aware that this important nerve lies very close to the anterolateral portal and that a protocolled arthroscopic technique can avoid injury to this structure.

It is fortunate that this nerve is visible on clinical examination (it is the only nerve in the body that can be seen in this way) [47]. By performing inversion of the ankle, the nerve is tensed (particularly the intermediate dorsal cutaneous branch), and its subcutaneous course becomes evident (see Fig. 3) [2]. Another means to achieve this end was reported by Stephens and Kelly [47], who proposed flexion of the fourth toe to accentuate the subcutaneous course of the dividing branches of the superficial peroneal nerve. A vertical incision affecting only the skin, together with blunt dissection up to the capsule, contributes to decreasing the risk of injury to the nerve. The anterolateral portal can also be created by an inside-out technique through the anteromedial portal, similar to the way the anterior portal is made in arthroscopy of the shoulder. Cutaneous transillumination obtained in this manner allows localization of the superficial peroneal nerve (intermediate dorsal cutaneous nerve) [5,48].

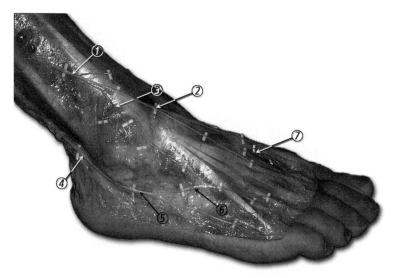

Fig. 8. Anatomic dissection of the cutaneous nerves at the dorsum of the foot. 1, superficial peroneal nerve; 2, medial dorsal cutaneous nerve; 3, intermediate dorsal cutaneous nerve; 4, sural
nerve; 5, lateral dorsal cutaneous nerve (terminal branch of sural nerve); 6, communication between
intermediate and lateral dorsal cutaneous nerve; 7, deep peroneal nerve.

Anterocentral portal

The anterocentral portal is established between the extensor digitorum longus
tendons at the level of the joint line. This portal provides a wide field of view
and facilitates passage of the instruments in the anteroposterior direction [21].
Nevertheless, most investigators discourage the use of this portal because there
is a high associated risk of injury to numerous neurovascular structures. These
structures include the medial dorsal cutaneous nerve (medial branch of the
superficial peroneal nerve), which runs subcutaneously, and the deep peroneal
nerve and the anterior tibial and dorsalis pedis arteries and veins, which are
found lying on the joint capsule (see Figs. 4 and 5). The fact that these structures are in such close relationship to the capsule justifies the potential for injury to the anterior tibial or dorsalis pedis artery (pseudoaneurysm). Injury does
not occur because the central portal is used for access but occurs when tibial
osteophytes are removed or when an anterior synovectomy is performed through
the anteromedial and anterolateral portals [49–51]. Moreover, anatomic variations in the course of the anterior tibial artery at the ankle may lead to vascular lesions [52,53]. Lateral deviation of this vessel, placing it in front of the
tibiofibular syndesmosis, has been found in 5.5% of patients (Fig. 9) [54]. This
possibility has made some investigators recommend the use of Doppler ultrasound at the joint line to localize the anterior tibial or dorsalis pedis artery
[52,53].

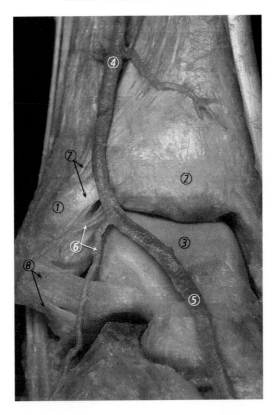

Fig. 9. Anatomic dissection showing varying course of the anterior tibial artery (lateral deviation). 1, lateral malleolus; 2, tibia; 3, talus; 4, anterior tibial artery; 5, dorsalis pedis artery; 6, anterior malleolar artery; 7, anterior tibiofibular ligament; 8, anterior talofibular ligament.

Medial midline portal

The medial midline portal was first described by Buckingham and colleagues [18], with the aim of obtaining an interarticular view similar to that of the anterocentral portal but with a lower risk of lesion to vital structures. The portal is located just lateral to the tibialis anterior tendon, between the tibialis anterior and the extensor hallucis longus tendon, which is located medial to the portal. This approach can also be used to introduce fluid into the joint.

Accessory portals

Additional portals can be performed proximal to the anterolateral and anteromedial portals. The separation between the main portal and the accessory portal should be wide enough to allow proper triangulation and instrumentation and to avoid the risk of cutaneous necrosis.

These portals can facilitate the instrumentation in certain diseases or can be used to introduce fluid into the joint.

Posterior portals

Because of the anteroposterior convexity of the joint, the posterior joint line is located 4 to 6 mm distal to the anterior joint line and is a difficult landmark to palpate. According to Guhl [39], the posterior joint line can be determined externally and is located 0.5 cm above the tip of the medial malleolus and 1 cm from the tip of the lateral malleolus. The authors do not favor use of the metric system for determining the position of the portals, although it can be useful in some cases. The authors prefer to use a spinal needle inserted under arthroscopic observation through the anterior portals to identify the joint line and determine proper positioning of the entrance point.

Posterolateral portal

The posterolateral is the most widely used of the posterior portals because it presents the lowest risk of neurovascular injury. It is located 1.2 to 2.5 cm proximal to the tip of the lateral malleolus, adjacent to the lateral axis of the Achilles tendon [2]. The sural nerve and its branches and the small saphenous vein are in close proximity and at risk of injury (Fig. 10) [5,21,42]. Ferkel and colleagues [5] reported five cases of sural nerve lesion in 612 arthroscopic procedures of the ankle. According to Feiwell and Frey [30], the sural nerve is

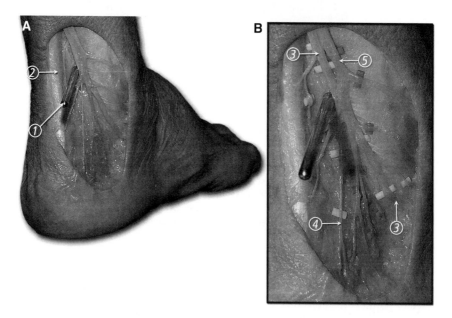

Fig. 10. (*A*) Anatomic dissection showing neurovascular relationships from the posterolateral portal. 1, Wissinger rod located in the posterolateral portal; 2, lateral border of calcaneal tendon. (*B*) Macrophotography. 3, sural nerve; 4, lateral calcaneal nerve (collateral branch of sural nerve); 5, small saphenous vein and branches.

located at a mean distance of 6 mm (0–12 mm) and the small saphenous vein at 9.5 mm (2–18 mm) from the posterolateral portal.

This portal is usually made with an outside-in technique. It is also possible to use an inside-out technique for this purpose [55], but considerable articular distraction is required to overcome the difference in positioning of the two joint lines, necessary for anteroposterior passage of the instruments.

In any case, after meticulous anatomic study of the posterior ligaments of the ankle joint [56] and having performed and observed numerous arthroscopic procedures in this articulation, the authors concluded that the posterolateral portal is always established between two posterior ligaments of the ankle joint—the transverse ligament and the posterior intermalleolar ligament—which are con-

A   **B**

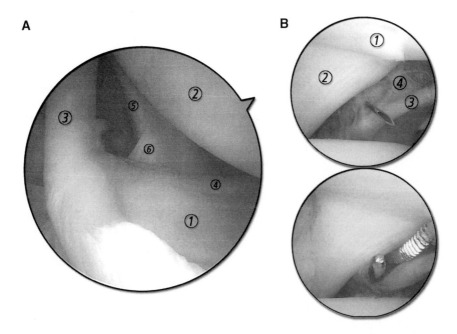

Fig. 11. (*A*) Arthroscopic image of the right shoulder through the anterior portal. Matthews and colleagues [57] described an intra-articular anatomic triangle used as a landmark to safely establish the anterior portal in shoulder arthroscopy. The triangle is delineated by the following: 1, glenoid cavity; 2, humeral head; and 3, long biceps brachii tendon; 4, anterior labrum; 5, subscapularis tendon; 6, middle glenohumeral ligament. (*B*) Ankle arthroscopy images (Courtesy of Prof. Pier Paolo Mariani, Department of Sports Traumatology, IUSM, University of Motor Sciences, Rome, Italy) of the posterior ligaments of the ankle through the anterolateral portal. Upper panel: 21-gauge needle inserted in optimal location of the posterolateral portal. Lower panel: Mosquito clamp used to open joint capsule before introducing cannula. 1, tibia; 2, medial border of the transverse ligament (deep component of the posterior tibiofibular ligament); 3, lateral border of the posterior intermalleolar ligament or tibial slip; 4, the triangular area where the posterolateral portal is usually created (delimited by the medial border of the transverse ligament and the posterior intermalleolar ligament, with the base at the tibia). The triangle is visible when the ankle is in dorsiflexion; the posterior intermalleolar ligament tenses and a gap is created between the intermalleolar and transverse ligaments.

stant and visible by arthroscopy. In dorsiflexion, the arrangement of these ligaments, together with the tibia, delimits a triangular area, with the base at the tibia and the tip at the lateral malleolus [56]. This space is similar to the anatomic intra-articular triangle of the shoulder used as a landmark to safely establish the anterior portal, as described by Matthews and colleagues [57] (Fig. 11).

TransAchilles portal

The transAchilles portal was described by Voto and colleagues [16] to obtain a wide field of view in the posterior compartment of the joint. It is established through the calcaneal tendon at the posterior joint line. This portal is not commonly used and has been discouraged by some investigators such as Ferkel and colleagues [2,5,15] because of the limited mobility of the instruments, the morbidity to the calcaneal tendon, and the potential for injury to the flexor hallucis longus tendon [15].

Posteromedial portal

The posteromedial portal is located adjacent to the medial axis of the calcaneal tendon. As occurs with the anterocentral portal, the use of this access route is not recommended because of the elevated risk of injury to several structures including the tibial nerve, the posterior tibial artery and veins, the flexor digitorum longus tendons, and the flexor hallucis longus tendon [15].

Posterior endoscopic portals

Even though numerous portals for accessing the ankle joint have been described and there are several available systems of distraction, the morphology of the joint makes access to the posterior region from the anterior portals difficult. For this reason and with the aim of resolving treatment of periarticular pathology, van Dijk and colleagues [19] described two posterior endoscopic portals that allow better access to the posterior ankle joint regions: the posterior aspect of the ankle joint and the subtalar joint.

To use these portals, the patient must be in the prone position, whereas for the portals described up to now, the patient is in the supine position (Fig. 12). As the authors understand it, van Dijk and colleagues [19] perform a modification of the method for establishing the conventional lateral and medial posterior portals, providing the possibility to treat periarticular pathology without necessarily accessing the articular space and considerably decreasing the risk of neurovascular lesions. By means of this technique, it is possible to inspect and treat lesions in the posterior part of the ankle joint and pathology in the subtalar joint. Among 86 consecutive endoscopic procedures performed, the investigators had no complications.

The posterolateral portal is created at the same level as or slightly above the tip of the lateral malleolus, just lateral to the calcaneal tendon. A blunt dissection is performed with a vascular or mosquito clamp, and the arthroscope shaft with a blunt trocar is inserted in the direction of the webspace between the first and second toe until it touches the talar bone (see Fig. 12A).

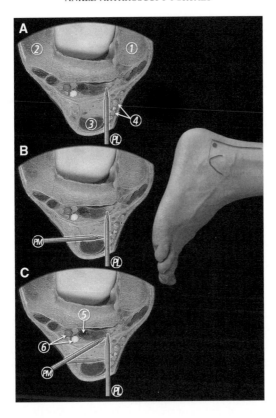

Fig. 12. (A–C) Macrophotography of a transverse section at the ankle joint. To show the anatomic relationships of the posterior portals, the arthroscopic cannulas have been added digitally (Adobe Photoshop). PL, posterolateral portal; PM, posteromedial portal; 1, lateral malleolus; 2, medial malleolus; 3, calcaneal tendon; 4, sural nerve and small saphenous vein; 5, flexor hallucis tendon (musculotendinous); 6, tibial nerve and posterior tibial artery and veins.

Subsequently, the posteromedial portal is established at the medial edge of the calcaneal tendon, at the same height as the posterolateral portal. The direction of the portal is the most important aspect to consider. The mosquito clamp is introduced and then arthroscope shaft with the blunt trocar is inserted in a medial-to-lateral direction until it touches the arthroscope shaft positioned in the posterolateral portal (see Fig. 12B). It then slides along the shaft, which acts as a guide, until the tip is reached (see Fig. 12C). After the periarticular fatty tissue is removed, the flexor hallucis longus tendon, the lateral talar process, the ankle joint capsule with the posterior ligaments of the joint, and the subtalar joint capsule can be identified. Among these structures, the flexor hallucis longus tendon acquires special relevance because the tibial neurovascular bundle (tibial nerve, posterior tibial artery and veins) is located medial to it (see Fig. 12). Care should be taken to avoid injury to the flexor hallucis longus tendon, which is considered the main endoscopic landmark because its lateral border determines

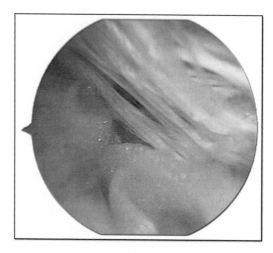

Fig. 13. Endoscopic image of the deep crural fascia with a transverse course and a consistent appearance.

the working area. Proper positioning of the ankle and the hallux results in better visualization of the tendinous portion of the flexor hallucis longus muscle and avoids unnecessary resection of some of the muscle fibers that reach the lateral tendinous border in a semipeniform morphology. Plantar flexion of the ankle or hallux flexion facilitates visualization of the flexor hallucis longus tendon proximal to the lateral talar process.

During resection of the periarticular fatty tissue, fascial fibers that have a transverse course and a consistent appearance can easily be recognized. These fibers are part of the deep crural fascia that, because of its constant movement, is considerably thickened at the level of the ankle joint. In 1932, Rouvière and Canela [58] gave this structure the name fibulotalocalcaneal ligament (Fig. 13).

The growing interest in the development and clinical application [34,35] of these two portals prompted Lijoi and colleagues [34,37] and Sitler and colleagues [36] to perform anatomic studies to verify the safety of their use relative to the structures susceptible to injury (the tibial nerve and the posterior tibial artery and veins); the investigators concluded that both portals are safe.

Summary

Although a large number of portals have been described, in most cases, only three—the anteromedial, the anterolateral, and the posterolateral—are required to perform diagnostic and therapeutic arthroscopy.

According to the recommendations of van Dijk and colleagues [59–61], clinicians should consider abandoning simultaneous use of anterior and posterior portals because of the difficulty involved in performing this combined technique that increases the risk of injury to vascular structures [36]. Given that it is diagnostic suspicion supported by numerous complementary examinations that determines the indication for arthroscopy, it seems reasonable to adopt a separation of arthroscopic pathology of the ankle into anterior compartment pathology and posterior compartment pathology [59–61]. Similarly, such diagnostic suspicion helps to determine whether there is a need to use distraction. The authors believe that the contribution of van Dijk and colleagues [59–61] in the use of distraction systems follows clear anatomical logic.

The ankle joint capsule is similar to the capsule of any other joint, with the exception of a singular characteristic: the anterior capsular insertion in the tibia and talus occurs at a distance from the cartilaginous layer. According to Testut and Latarjet [62], the distance is approximately 6 to 8 mm in the tibia and 8 to 10 mm in the talus. In a recent study, the distance was found to be 4.3 mm (0.5–9.0 mm) and 2.4 mm (1.8–3.3 mm) in the tibia and talus, respectively [63]. This peculiarity determines the existence of a substantial anterior capsular recess that allows the arthroscopist to encounter a working area. Nevertheless, the size of this area depends on the position of the foot. When the foot is in dorsiflexion, the capsular recess is evident, whereas when it is in plantar flexion, capsular tension makes the recess smaller. Hence, van Dijk and colleagues [64] recommended that treatment of anterior pathology should be done with the joint in dorsiflexion: "the anterior working area is opened up and a bony or soft tissue impediment in front of the malleolus, at the talar neck or at the distal tibia can be visualised and treated." Moreover, when the joint is in dorsiflexion, the talus is protected within the articulation, and the risk of injury to the cartilage when creating the anterior portals is minimized. Similarly, when distraction is

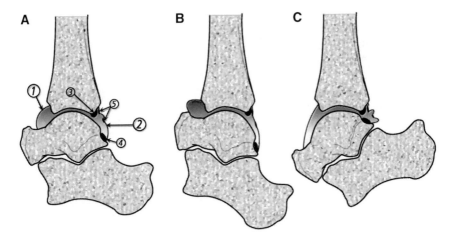

Fig. 14. (*A*) Schematic view of the ankle joint at 90° and the anterior working area. 1, anterior capsular joint; 2, posterior capsular joint; 3, transverse ligament or deep component of posterior tibiofibular ligament; 4, posterior talofibular ligament; 5, posterior intermalleolar ligament. (*B*) The anterior working area is opened in dorsiflexion of the foot; anterior impingement can easily be treated. (*C*) When the foot is in plantar flexion, the anterior working area is reduced.

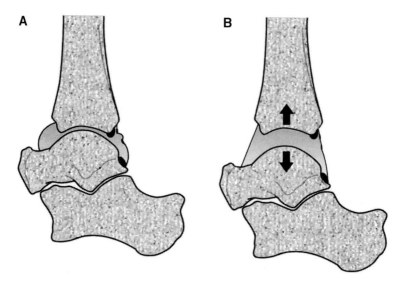

Fig. 15. (*A*) Schematic view of the ankle joint at 90° showing the anterior and posterior anterior and posterior working areas. (*B*) Interarticular work is possible when distraction (*arrows*) is used, but the capsular tension reduces the anterior and posterior working areas.

used, the tension in the articular capsule is increased and applied to the bone ends, reducing the working area (Fig. 14).

If we transfer these concepts to the posterior compartment and to the use of the classic posterolateral portal, there are some differences. In contrast to what occurs with the anterior portal, the posterior articular recess is smaller, and the presence of structures that reinforce the capsule, such as the posterior intermalleolar ligament or tibial slip, convert it into multiple small recesses, making interarticular positioning of the arthroscope or instrumentation difficult in the posterolateral portal. In addition, when a distraction system is applied, capsular tension reduces the working space even more. Thus, the authors believe that the classic posterolateral portal does not provide any relevant advantage (Fig. 15).

Acknowledgments

The authors thank Celine Cavallo for the English translation of the text.

References

[1] Pena Gómez FA, Amendola N. The ankle. In: McGuinty J, editor. Operative arthroscopy. 3rd edition. Philadelphia: JB Lippincott Williams & Wilkins; 2003. p. 187–9.
[2] Ferkel RD. Arthroscopic surgery. The foot and ankle. Philadelphia: Lippincot-Raven; 1996.

[3] Zini R. Artroscopia della caviglia. Manuale pratico di tecnica chuirurgica [Arthroscopy of the ankle. Practical manual of the surgical technique]. Fano: Editrice Fortuna; 1996 [in Italian].

[4] Burman MS. Arthroscopy or the direct visualization of joints. An experimental cadaver study. Am J Bone Joint Surg 1931;13:669–95.

[5] Ferkel RD, Guhl JF, Heath DD. Neurological complications of ankle arthroscopy. Arthroscopy 1996;12(35):200–8.

[6] Watanabe M. Selfoc-Arthroscopy (Watanabe no. 24 arthroscope). Monograph. Tokyo: Teishin Hospital; 1972.

[7] Ikehuchi H. Arthroscopy of the ankle. Presented at the International Arthroscopy Association Meeting. 1977.

[8] Chen YC. Clinical and cadaver studies on the ankle joint arthroscopy. J Jpn Orthop Assoc 1976; 50:631–51.

[9] Drez D, Guhl JF, Gollehon DL. Ankle arthroscopy: technique and indications. Foot Ankle 1981;2:138–43.

[10] Drez Jr D, Guhl JF, Gollehon DL. Ankle arthroscopy: technique and indications. Clin Sports Med 1982;1:35–45.

[11] Parisien JS, Shereff MJ. The role of arthroscopy in the diagnosis and treatment of disorders of the ankle. Foot Ankle 1981;2:144–9.

[12] Parisien JS, Vangsness T. Operative arthroscopy of the ankle. Three years' experience. Clin Orthop Rel Res 1985;199:46–53.

[13] Parisien JS, Vangsness T, Feldman R. Diagnostic and operative arthroscopy of the ankle. An experimental approach. Clin Orthop Rel Res 1987;224:228–36.

[14] Andrews JR, Previte WJ, Carson WG. Arthroscopy of the ankle: technique and normal anatomy. Foot Ankle 1985;6:29–33.

[15] Ferkel RD, Fischer SP. Progress in ankle arthroscopy. Clin Orthop Rel Res 1989;240:210–20.

[16] Voto SJ, Ewing JW, Fleissner PR, et al. Ankle arthroscopy: neurovascular and arthroscopic anatomy of standard and trans-Achilles tendon portal placement. Arthroscopy 1989;5:41–6.

[17] Mandrino A, Chabaud B, Moyen B, et al. Arthroscopie de la cheville: un nouveau point d'entrée postéro-interne. Note de technique [Arthroscopy of the ankle: a new postero-internal point of entry. Technical note]. Rev Chir Orthop 1994;80:342–5 [in French].

[18] Buckingham RA, Winson IG, Kelly AJ. An anatomical study of a new portal for ankle arthroscopy. J Bone Joint Surg Br 1997;79:650–2.

[19] van Dijk CN, Scholten PE, Krips R. A 2-portal endoscopic approach for diagnosis and treatment of posterior ankle pathology. Technical note. Arthroscopy 2000;16:871–6.

[20] Acevedo JI, Busch MT, Ganey TM, et al. Coaxial portals for posterior ankle arthroscopy: an anatomic study with clinical correlation on 29 patients. Arthroscopy 2000;16:836–42.

[21] Guhl JF. New concepts (distraction) in ankle arthroscopy. Arthroscopy 1988;4:160–7.

[22] Yates CK, Grana WA. A simple distraction technique for ankle arthroscopy. Arthroscopy 1988; 4:103–5.

[23] Trager S, Frederick LD, Seligson D. Ankle arthroscopy. Orthopaedics 1989;12:1317–20.

[24] Casteleyn PP, Handelberg F. A simple distraction technique for ankle arthroscopy. J Bone Joint Surg Br 1993;75(Suppl II):138.

[25] Kumar VP, Satku K. The A-O femoral distractor for ankle arthroscopy. Technical note. Arthroscopy 1994;10:118–9.

[26] Casteleyn PP, Handelberg F. Distraction for ankle arthroscopy. Technical note. Arthroscopy 1995;11:633–4.

[27] Sartoretti C, Sartoretti-Schefer S, Duff C, Buchmann P. Angioplasty balloon catheters used for distraction of the ankle joint. Arthroscopy 1996;12:82–6.

[28] Cameron SE. Noninvasive distraction for ankle arthroscopy. Technical note. Arthroscopy 1997;13:366–9.

[29] van Dijk CN, Verhagen RAW, Tol HJL. Resterilizable noninvasive ankle distraction device. Technical note. Arthroscopy 2001;17:e1–5.

[30] Feiwell LA, Frey C. Anatomic study of arthroscopic portal sites of the ankle. Foot Ankle 1993; 14:142–7.

[31] Takao M, Uchio Y, Shu N, et al. Anatomic bases of ankle arthroscopy: study of superficial and deep peroneal nerves around anterolateral and anterocentral approach. Surg Radiol Anat 1998;20:317–20.

[32] Saito A, Kikuchi S. Anatomic relations between ankle arthroscopic portal sites and the superficial peroneal and saphenous nerves. Foot Ankle 1998;19:748–52.

[33] Ögüt T, Akgüm H, Kesmezacar H, et al. Pathology of the posterior compartment of the ankle: Arthroscopic treatment by the posterior approach. Surg Radiol Anat 2004;26:268–74.

[34] Lijoi F, Lughi M, Baccarani G. Patologia del comparto posteriore della caviglia: Trattamento artroscopico per via posteriore. Artroscopia 2002;3:30–5 [in Italian].

[35] Lohrer H, Arentz S. Posterior approach for arthroscopic treatment of posterolateral impingement syndrome of the ankle in a top-level field hockey player. Arthroscopy 2004;20:e15–21.

[36] Sitler DF, Amendola A, Bailey CS, et al. Posterior ankle arthroscopy: an anatomic study. J Bone Joint Surg Am 2002;84:763–9.

[37] Lijoi F, Lughi M, Baccarani G. Posterior arthroscopic approach to the ankle: an anatomic study. Arthroscopy 2003;19:62–7.

[38] Harty M. Ankle arthroscopy, anatomical features. Orthopaedics 1985;8:1538–40.

[39] Ghul JF. Foot and ankle arthroscopy. 2nd edition. New York: Slack Inc.; 1993.

[40] Reinmann R. Der variable Streckapparat der Kleinen Zehe [Variations in the extensor apparatus of the fifth toe]. Gegenbaurs Morphol Jahrb 1981;127:188–209 [in German].

[41] Takao M, Ochi M, Shu N, et al. A case of superficial peroneal nerve injury during ankle arthroscopy. Arthroscopy 2001;17:403–4.

[42] Martin DF, Baker CL, Curl WW, et al. Operative ankle arthroscopy. Am J Sports Med 1989; 17:16–23.

[43] Barber FA, Click J, Britt BT. Complications of ankle arthroscopy. Foot Ankle 1990;10:263–6.

[44] Adkison DP, Bosse MJ, Gaccione DR, et al. Anatomic variations in the course of the superficial peroneal nerve. J Bone Joint Surg Am 1991;73:112–4.

[45] Blair JM, Botte MJ. Surgical anatomy of the superficial peroneal nerve in the ankle and foot. Clin Orthop Rel Res 1994;305:229–38.

[46] Sayli U, Tekdemyr Y, Cubuk HE, et al. The course of the superficial peroneal nerve: an anatomical cadáver study. Foot Ankle Surg 1998;4:63–9.

[47] Stephens MM, Kelly PM. Fourth toe in flexion sign: a new clinical sign for identification of the superficial nerve. Foot Ankle Int 2000;21:860–3.

[48] Barber FA, Britt BT, Ratliff HW, et al. Arthroscopy surgery of the ankle. Orthop Rev 1988; 17:446–51.

[49] O'Farrell D, Dudeney S, McNally S, et al. Pseudoaneurysm formation after ankle arthroscopy. Foot Ankle 1997;18:578–9.

[50] Salgado CJ, Mukherjee D, Quist MA, et al. Anterior tibial artery pseudoaneurysm after ankle arthroscopy. Cardiovasc Surg 1998;6:604–6.

[51] Mariani PP, Mancini L, Giorgini T. Pseudoaneurysm as a complication of ankle arthroscopy. Case report. Arthroscopy 2001;17:400–2.

[52] Golanó P, Forcada P, Carrera A, et al. Arterias potencialmente lesionables durante la artroscopia de tobillo [Arteries at risk of injury during ankle arthroscopy]. Cuadernos de Artroscopia 1996; 3:50–7 [in Spanish].

[53] Darwish A, Ehsan O, Marynissen H, et al. Pseudoaneurysm of the anterior tibial artery after ankle arthroscopy. Case report. Arthroscopy 2004;20:E13.

[54] Huber JF. The arterial network supplying the dorsum of the foot. Anat Rec 1941;80:373–91.

[55] Katchis SD, Smith RW. A simple way to establish the posterolateral portal in ankle arthroscopy. Technique tip. Foot Ankle 1997;18:178–9.

[56] Golanó P, Mariani PP, Rodríguez-Niedenfuhr M, et al. Arthroscopic anatomy of the posterior ankle ligaments. Arthroscopy 2002;18:353–8.

[57] Matthews LS, Zarins B, Michael RH, et al. Anterior portal selection for shoulder arthroscopy. Arthroscopy 1985;1:33–9.

[58] Rouvière H, Canela M. Le ligament peronéo-astragalo-calacanéen [The fibulotalocalcaneal ligament]. Ann Anat Pathol (Paris) 1932;9:745–50 [in French].

[59] van Dijk CN, Tol JL, Verheyen CCPM. A prospective study of prognostic factors concerning the outcome of arthroscopic surgery for anterior ankle impingement. Am J Sports Med 1997;25: 737–45.

[60] Van Dijk CN. Arthroscopy of the ankle. Arthroscopy 1997;13:90–6.

[61] Van Dijk CN. Ankle joint arthroscopy. Surg Tech Orthop Traumatol 2001;55(630):A10.

[62] Testut L, Latarjet A. Anatomia humana, vol 1. [A treatise on human anatomy]. Barcelona, Spain: Salvat Editores; 1985 [in Spanish].

[63] Tol JL, van Dijk CN. Etiology of the anterior ankle impingement syndrome: a descriptive anatomical study. Foot Ankle Int 2004;25:382–6.

[64] Van Dijk CN, Bossuyt PM, Marti RK. Medial ankle pain after lateral ligament rupture. J Bone Joint Surg Br 1996;78:562–7.

ELSEVIER
SAUNDERS

Foot Ankle Clin N Am
11 (2006) 275–296

FOOT AND
ANKLE CLINICS

Ankle Anatomy for the Arthroscopist. Part II: Role of the Ankle Ligaments in Soft Tissue Impingement

Pau Golanó, MD[a],*, Jordi Vega, MD[a,b],
Luis Pérez-Carro, MD, PhD[c], Víctor Götzens, MD, PhD[a]

[a]*Laboratory of Arthroscopic and Surgical Anatomy, Department of Pathology and
Experimental Therapeutics (Human Anatomy Unit), University of Barcelona,
c/ Feixa Llarga s/n (Campus Bellvitge), L'Hospitalet de Llobregat, Barcelona 08907, Spain*
[b]*Department of Orthopedic and Trauma Surgery, "La Mútua," Granollers, Barcelona, Spain*
[c]*Department of Orthopedic and Trauma Surgery, Centro Médico Lealtad, Santander, Spain*

Injury to the ankle ligaments is one of the leading sports injuries. Lesions affecting the ankle are more frequent in sports such as basketball (45%), handball (25%), and soccer (31%) [1]. Nevertheless, there are relatively few published studies centering on these ligaments compared with other joints such as the cruciate ligaments of the knee.

Together with the joint capsule and the retinacula, the ankle ligaments are important static stabilizers. In the lateral and medial areas of the joint, they are grouped into two large ligamentous complexes under the names lateral collateral ligament (LCL) and medial collateral ligament (MCL) or deltoid ligament.

The most common mechanism of injury to the ankle ligaments is inversion of the foot. This mechanism affects 75% [2] to over 90% [3] of the cases involving the LCL, and particularly one of its elements, the anterior talofibular ligament. Injury to the MCL is much less frequent, accounting for about 15% of all ligamentous lesions [4]. MCL injury rarely occurs alone; it is more often associated with other ligamentous injuries or with fractures. Syndesmotic injuries occur in 1% to 18% [5] of patients who have an ankle sprain and are more common in collision sports.

* Corresponding author.
E-mail address: pgolano@ub.edu (P. Golanó).

1083-7515/06/$ – see front matter © 2006 Elsevier Inc. All rights reserved.
doi:10.1016/j.fcl.2006.03.003

foot.theclinics.com

Following an ankle sprain, 10% to 50% of patients present with some kind of chronic pain. The most frequent cause of chronic pain after an ankle sprain is known as soft tissue impingement syndrome [1], and the primary etiology of this condition is injury to the ligamentous structures. Therefore, an understanding of the anatomy and biomechanics of the ligamentous complexes is essential for diagnosis and adequate treatment of this condition.

To simplify the description of the ankle ligaments, this article is divided into two sections: (1) the ligaments that join the distal epiphyses of the bones of the leg (tibia and fibula): the ligaments of the distal tibiofibular syndesmosis; and (2) the ligaments that join the tibia and fibula to the skeletal structure of the foot: the LCL and MCL.

Ligaments that join the distal epiphyses of the tibia and fibula

The distal epiphyses of the tibia and fibula are firmly joined by ligaments that make up a moveable joint system encompassing the talus, thus forming the talocrural joint. The articular surfaces of the tibia and the fibula form a triangular configuration with a proximal base. The surface provided by the fibula and the tibia, called the tibial and fibular notch, respectively, is rough in the proximal region because it is the insertion site for one of the syndesmotic ligaments (the interosseous tibiofibular ligament), which is simply the continuation of the interosseous membrane at this level. Distal to the insertion site of this ligament, the remaining anterior surface corresponds to the tibiofibular synovial recess of the ankle joint, and at the posterior surface, there is a small bundle of adipose tissue called the fatty synovial fringe (Fig. 1). The synovial fringe lowers or rises during ankle movements, retracting in dorsiflexion to rise and to position itself between the tibia and fibula and descending in plantar flexion toward the ankle joint [6]. This structure has been implicated as a cause of chronic pain following ankle sprain in the condition known as anterolateral soft tissue impingement [7] or, more specifically, syndesmotic impingement [8,9].

As can be deduced from the previous description, the distal tibiofibular joint has no articular cartilage. It is a syndesmotic articulation that allows the tibia/fibula as a whole to adapt to the varying width of the upper articular surface of the talus by slight ascending and medial rotation movements of the fibula during extreme dorsiflexion (maximum width) and by inverse movements during plantar flexion (minimum width) [10].

Three ligaments join the distal tibial and fibular epiphyses: the anterior or anteroinferior tibiofibular ligament, the posterior or posteroinferior tibiofibular ligament, and the interosseous tibiofibular ligament. The inferior segment of the interosseous membrane also helps stabilize the tibiofibular syndesmosis.

Most anatomy books provide only a brief description of these ligaments. The related clinical studies also fail to describe them in detail, with the investigators mainly citing information found in other articles or anatomy books. There are also problems related to the terms used for the ligaments. For example, the

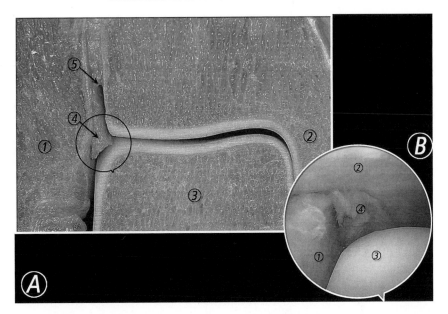

Fig. 1. Anatomic–arthroscopic correlation. (*A*) Frontal section of the ankle joint at the posterior region of the tibiofibular syndesmosis. 1, lateral malleolus; 2, tibia; 3, talus; 4, synovial fringe; 5, tibiofibular synovial recess. (*B*) Arthroscopic view of the synovial fringe through the anterolateral portal. 1, lateral malleolus; 2, plantar articular surface of the tibia; 3, dorsal articular surface of the talus; 4, synovial fringe.

official book of anatomic terminology [11] omits the interosseous tibiofibular ligament, as do many of the anatomy books the authors consulted. A similar problem is seen with the terms used for the other two syndesmotic ligaments that stabilize the proximal epiphyses of the tibia and fibula: the anterior and posterior tibiofibular ligaments [12], and the posterior tibiofibular ligament has been given a variety of names (see the Posterior or Posteroinferior Tibiofibular Ligament section).

Anterior or anteroinferior tibiofibular ligament

The anterior tibiofibular ligament is the weakest of all the syndesmotic ligaments, and the first to yield when the fibula is turned outward over its longitudinal axis [13]. The ligament originates in the anterior margin of the lateral malleolus and its fibers extend in a proximal and medial direction to the insertion site in the anterior tubercle of the tibia, with increases in the length of the fibers distally. On examination, the ligament is seen to be divided into several fascicles, which gives it a multifascicular morphology (Fig. 2). This multifascicular appearance is probably due to its relationship with the perforating branch of the peroneal artery, which runs along the surface of the ligament and provides small

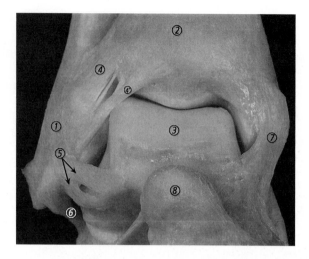

Fig. 2. Anatomic view of the anterior ligaments of the ankle. 1, lateral malleolus; 2, tibia; 3, talus; 4, anterior tibiofibular ligament; 4′, distal fascicle of the anterior tibiofibular ligament; 5, anterior talofibular ligament; 6, calcaneofibular ligament; 7, superficial and deep layers of the MCL; 8, head of the talus.

vessels that penetrate through the interfascicular spaces. The most distal fibers of the ligament at its origin may be confused with those of the anterior talofibular ligament [14–16].

On careful inspection, the most distal fascicle of the anterior tibiofibular ligament appears to be independent from the rest of the structure. It is separated by a septum of fibroadipose tissue and may be slightly deeper than the rest of the ligament. In its oblique course toward insertion in the tibia, the fascicle covers the angle formed by the tibia and fibula and comes into contact with the dorsolateral border of the talus during flexion of the ankle (see Fig. 2; Fig. 3). Knowledge of this configuration is important to understand the anatomic bases for anterolateral soft tissue impingement [16] because abrasion between the distal fascicle of the anterior tibiofibular ligament and the talus may lead to pain.

This relative independence of the distal fascicle from the anterior tibiofibular ligament led investigators such as Nikolopoulos [17] to give it a separate name: the accessory anteroinferior tibiofibular ligament. This term was refuted years later by Bassett and colleagues [15] following an anatomic study of 11 cadaver ankles, which led to its designation as distal fascicle of the anteroinferior tibiofibular ligament. Bassett and colleagues [15] measured the dimensions and the degrees of dorsiflexion needed for the distal fascicle to come into contact with the talus (mean, 12°) and observed that the fascicle has an intracapsular and extrasynovial location, thereby explaining why it can be seen by arthroscopy. These researchers also published a series of seven case studies in which resection of the distal fascicle of the anterior tibiofibular ligament satisfactorily resolved the symptoms of patients who had chronic ankle pain and a history of inversion

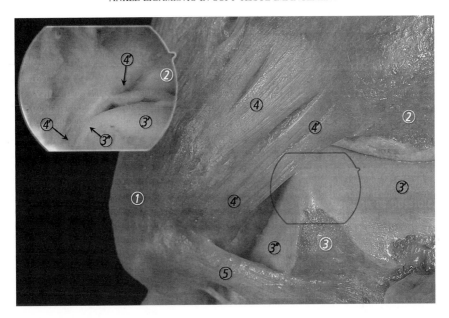

Fig. 3. Anatomic–arthroscopic correlation showing contact between the talus and the distal fascicle of the anterior tibiofibular ligament. The most distal fascicle of the anterior tibiofibular ligament appears to be independent from the rest of the structure and comes into contact with the dorsolateral border of the talus. 1, lateral malleolus; 2, tibia; 3, talus (beveled triangular region); 3′, dorsal articular surface of the talus; 3″, lateral or malleolar articular surface of the talus; 4, anterior tibiofibular ligament; 4′, distal fascicle of the anterior tibiofibular ligament; 5, anterior talofibular ligament.

sprains of the ankle. Thickening of the ligament was seen in all cases; five patients additionally showed abrasion of the joint cartilage in the region where the ligament came into contact with the talus. Bassett and colleagues [15] were the first to mention ligamentous etiology as the cause of impingement in the English literature. Resection of the distal fascicle as a therapeutic approach, whether by open surgery or arthroscopy, does not produce noticeable changes in the stability of the ankle [15,17–19] and may lead to clinical improvement.

Impingement of the distal fascicle of the anterior tibiofibular ligament seems to depend on changes in the ankle mechanics [15]. An injury to the LCL (eg, anterior talofibular ligament) increases anteroposterior laxity of the ankle [20], which in turn results in increased anterior extrusion of the talus and causes the distal fascicle to have greater contact and pressure on the talus [15]. Another factor related to distal fascicle impingement is the level at which the anterior tibiofibular ligament is inserted in the fibula with respect to the joint line. More distal insertion of the ligament could lead to increased contact in the neutral position of the ankle and a higher potential for ligamentous pathology [21]. Subsequent to Bassett and colleagues' studies, the distal fascicle has been the subject of numerous publications that have provided further definition of the anatomy of this structure and correlations with impingement [12,16,21,22].

Ray and Kriz [22] defined anterior tibiofibular ligament variations and the relationships between this ligament and the talus, which were classified into five types (I–V). The incidence of distal fascicle was 21.7%. According to these investigators, the presence of a separate fascicle is not a requirement for impingement; however, a beveled triangular region in the anterior superolateral border of the talus is common. Akseki and colleagues [21] noted that the cartilage is usually of poorer quality in this area when there is impingement and reported that the incidence of a distal fascicle was approximately 91%. Nikolopoulos [18] observed the presence of a distal fascicle in 82.9% to 91.6% of the cases and continued to call it an accessory ligament. The differences in the reported incidence of this structure could be due considerations related to the strict definition of a separate fascicle.

The authors' observations in the dissection room have allowed them to identify contact between the distal fascicle and the talus in the neutral position. This finding is frequently observed during ankle arthroscopy, and surgeons should consider it a normal feature [21]. This fact has been reported by other investigators [16,18,22–24], although in cases of anatomic variation or ankle instability, the feature may be pathologic (Fig. 4). Contact decreases with joint

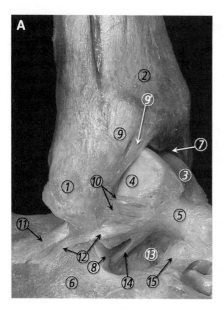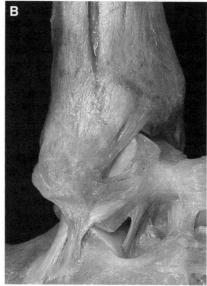

Fig. 4. Anatomic dissection (osteoarticular layer) showing the areas of contact between the talus and the distal fascicle of the anterior tibiofibular ligament, depending on the position of the ankle. (*A*) Ankle at 90°. 1, lateral malleolus (tip); 2, tibia; 3, dorsal articular surface of the talus; 4, lateral or malleolar articular surface of the talus; 5, neck of the talus; 6, calcaneus; 7, talocrural joint; 8, posterior subtalar joint; 9, anterior tibiofibular ligament; 9′, distal fascicle of the anterior tibiofibular ligament; 10, anterior talofibular ligament; 11, calcaneofibular ligament; 12, lateral talocalcaneal ligament; 13, tarsal sinus; 14, talocalcaneal interosseous ligament; 15, cervical ligament. (*B*) Ankle in dorsal flexion.

distraction [21], and this should be taken into account during arthroscopy. Akseki and colleagues [21] observed that section of the anterior talofibular ligament does not alter the contact when the ankle is in neutral position, although important changes are observed when the ankle is in movement, corroborating the theory proposed by Bassett and colleagues [15]. Therefore, ankle instability is one direct factor in anterior tibiofibular ligament pathology.

A diagnosis of this type of ligamentous impingement should be considered in patients who have chronic pain in the anterolateral area of the ankle following a sprain, joint stability, and a normal radiologic study [25]. Kim and Ha [26] considered that isolated impingement by this entity is uncommon, the condition usually being associated with hypertrophic scar tissue of the anterior talofibular ligament.

Posterior or posteroinferior tibiofibular ligament

According to the classic descriptions, the posterior or posteroinferior tibiofibular ligament is formed by two components, one superficial and the other deep [14], although this subdivision is not accepted by all investigators. Based on its position, Nikolopoulos [18] compared this ligament to the anterior tibiofibular ligament and its distal fascicle. The terminology used for this ligament and its components is controversial [12], which is particularly evident in the arthroscopic literature [27].

Superficial component

The superficial component originates at the posterior edge of the lateral malleolus and runs proximally and medially toward the tibia where it inserts in the posterior tubercle. This component would be homologous to the anterior tibiofibular ligament. The term posterior or posteroinferior tibiofibular ligament is usually used to refer to the superficial component.

Deep component

Sarrafian [14] coined the term *transverse ligament* to refer to the deep component. This structure is cone-shaped, turning on its fibers during its course. It originates in the proximal area of the malleolar fossa and runs toward the tibia, with insertion at the posterior edge of the tibia, immediately posterior to the cartilaginous covering of the inferior tibial articular surface; the fibers may reach the medial malleolus. The transverse ligament extends beyond the osseous margin in the distal direction and comprises a true labrum [14], which is dependent on the inferior articular surface of the tibia. By increasing the size and concavity of the tibial joint surface, the labrum provides talocrural joint stability and prevents posterior talar translation (Fig. 5) [28].

Because of its location and the limited joint surface provided by the lateral malleolus, the transverse ligament comes into contact with the talus. The inden-

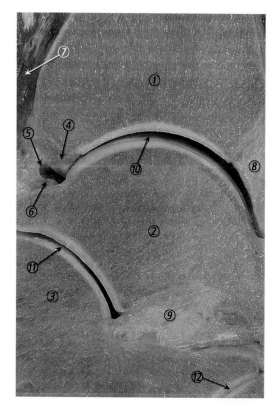

Fig. 5. Sagittal section of the ankle. 1, tibia; 2, talus; 3, calcaneus; 4, transverse ligament or deep component of the posterior tibiofibular ligament; 5, posterior capsular recess of the ankle joint; 6, posterior talofibular ligament; 7, flexor hallucis longus; 8, fatty tissue in the anterior capsular recess; 9, talocalcaneal interosseous ligament and tarsal sinus; 10, talocrural joint; 11, posterior sub-talar joint; 12, calcaneocuboid joint.

tation of this ligament in the talus results in a triangular surface with a posterior base at the lateral edge of the talar body in its posterior half [14].

On arthroscopic examination through anterior portals, many investigators report that the posterior tibiofibular ligament (superficial component) is readily visualized, but there is some controversy regarding the transverse ligament (deep component). The author and colleagues [27] have shown that only the deep component is visible arthroscopically and that the superficial component cannot be seen, thus helping to clarify previous descriptions of this ligament that may be confusing (Fig. 6).

Interosseous tibiofibular ligament

The interosseous tibiofibular ligament is a dense mass of short fibers that, together with adipose tissue and small branching vessels from the peroneal artery,

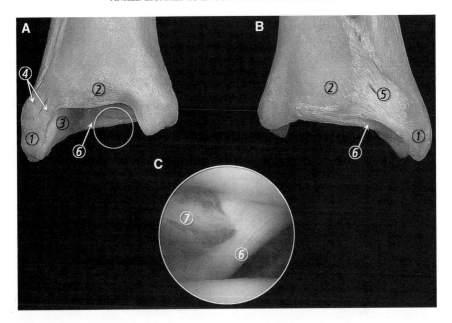

Fig. 6. (*A*) Anterior view, (*B*) posterior view, and (*C*) arthroscopic image (courtesy of Prof. Pier Paolo Mariani, Department of Sports Traumatology, IUSM, University of Motor Sciences, Rome, Italy) of the syndesmotic ligaments. 1, lateral malleolus (tip); 2, tibia; 3, malleolar articular surface; 4, anterior tibiofibular ligament; 5, superficial component of the posterior tibiofibular ligament; 6, transverse ligament or deep component of the posterior tibiofibular ligament.

span the tibia to the fibula. It can be considered a distal continuation of the interosseous membrane at the level of the tibiofibular syndesmosis [6,14].

Ligaments that join the leg bones to the skeletal structure of the foot

The ligaments that join the tibia and fibula to the skeletal structure of the foot have been grouped into two main ligamentous complexes, the LCL and the MCL.

Lateral collateral ligaments

Located on the lateral part of the joint, the LCL comprises three fascicles or ligaments, entirely independent of one another: the anterior talofibular, the calcaneofibular, and the posterior talofibular ligaments.

Anterior talofibular ligament

The anterior talofibular ligament is the most frequently injured ligament of the ankle. This flat, quadrilateral ligament is in close contact with the capsule and is typically composed of two bands separated by an interval that allows penetration of the vascular branches from the perforating peroneal artery and its anastomosis with the lateral malleolar artery; the upper band is larger than the lower one. Occasionally there are three bands [14], although the authors have never observed this morphology in their dissections. Milner and Soames [29] found that the ligament had a single band in 38% of cases, two bands in 50% of cases, and three bands in 12%, in contrast with Sarrafian's [14] observations. Nevertheless, it is notable that subsequent anatomic studies [30,31] to determine the anatomy and dimensions of the parts of the LCL do not stress this aspect. In a study using MRI to investigate 22 patients who had no history of ankle sprains, Delfaut and colleagues [32] found that the anterior talofibular ligament had a single band in 9% of cases, two bands in 55%, and a striated appearance in 36%. The authors' dissections have shown that this ligament most commonly has a double-band morphology, as described by Sarrafian [14]. The upper band reaches the origin of the anterior tibiofibular ligament, and the inferior band reaches the origin of the calcaneofibular ligament. In many specimens, these latter ligaments (talofibular and calcaneofibular ligament) are joined by arciform fibers at the malleolar origin (Fig. 7) [14].

In its entirety, the anterior talofibular ligament originates at the anterior margin of the lateral malleolus. From its origin, it runs anteromedially to the insertion

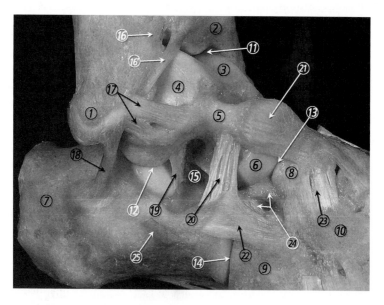

Fig. 7. Osteoarticular anatomic dissection of the ligaments of the foot and ankle joint. 1, lateral malleolus (tip); 2, tibia; 3, dorsal articular surface of the talus; 4, lateral or malleolar articular surface of the talus; 5, neck of the talus; 6, head of the talus; 7, calcaneus; 8, navicular; 9, cuboid; 10, lateral cuneiform; 11, talocrural joint; 12, posterior subtalar joint; 13, talonavicular joint; 14, calcaneocuboid joint; 15, tarsal sinus; 16, anterior tibiofibular ligament; 16′, distal fascicle of the anterior tibiofibular ligament; 17, anterior talofibular ligament; 18, calcaneofibular ligament; 19, talocalcaneal interosseous ligament; 20, cervical ligament; 21, talonavicular ligament; 22, lateral calcaneocuboid ligament; 23, dorsal cuneonavicular ligament; 24, bifurcate ligament; 25, peroneal tubercle.

points at the talus body immediately anterior to the joint surface occupied by the lateral malleolus and consists of two small tubercles visible in osseous anatomic preparations and corresponding to the insertion sites of each of the bands. The ligament is virtually horizontal to the ankle in the neutral position but inclines upward in dorsiflexion and downward in plantar flexion.

Ferkel and colleagues [33,34] cited this ligament as another cause of antero-lateral soft tissue impingement, indicating that although an injury to this ligament may not be severe enough to cause chronic instability, inadequate treatment could lead to an inflammatory process in the area of the injury, followed by synovitis and the formation of prominent scar tissue. This mass of tissue would occupy the lateral recess of the joint, possibly causing pain and irritation that would lead to the development of additional inflammatory tissue and eventually to chronic pain [33,34]. Chronic progression of this inflammatory tissue, together with remnant scar tissue, would produce the so-called "meniscoid tissue" described by Wolin and colleagues [35].

Calcaneofibular ligament

The calcaneofibular ligament is a thick, cordlike ligament that originates at the anterior edge of the lateral malleolus, right below the origin of the lower band of the anterior talofibular ligament, to which it can be joined by arciform fibers. It is important to note that the origin of this ligament does not reach the tip of the malleolus, which remains free from ligamentous insertions, as is observed during ankle arthroscopy. In the neutral position, the ligament courses backward, downward, and medially, and inserts in a small tubercle in the posterior region of the lateral calcaneus, posterior to the peroneal tubercle (see Fig. 7).

This ligament is superficially crossed by the peroneal tendons and sheaths, which can leave a concavity over the ligament; only about 1 cm of the ligament is uncovered [14]. In addition, the calcaneofibular ligament is separated from the subtalar (talocalcaneal) joint by the lateral talocalcaneal ligament, and is further separated from this ligament by adipose tissue. The anatomic variants of the calcaneofibular ligament and their relationship with the lateral talocalcaneal ligament have been the subject of study [36].

The calcaneofibular ligament controls two joints—the talocrural joint and the subtalar joint—unlike the other two elements making up the LCL, which only affect the talocrural. Little attention has been given to this ligament compared with the other ligaments of the LCL, although variants in the orientation of the structure have been studied by Ruth [37]. The calcaneofibular ligament becomes horizontal during extension and vertical in flexion, remaining tense throughout its entire arc of motion. A valgus or varus position of the talus considerably changes the angle formed by the ligament and the longitudinal axis of the fibula. The ligament is relaxed in the valgus position and tense in the varus position, which explains the potential for injury even without dorsiflexion/plantar flexion move-ment in the ankle.

According to Ferkel and colleagues [34], in cases in which injury to the anterior talofibular ligament is associated with injury to the calcaneofibular ligament, the latter also contributes to the development of anterolateral soft tissue impingement.

Posterior talofibular ligament

The posterior talofibular ligament is a strong, thick, fascicled, trapezoidal ligament in an intracapsular extrasynovial location, found in an almost horizontal plane. It originates on the medial surface of the lateral malleolus in the malleolar fossa and courses toward the posterolateral talus. The fibers of the ligament are inserted along the lateral aspect of the talus on a rough, grooved surface situated along the posteroinferior border of the talar lateral malleolar surface. Other fibers are inserted in the posterior surface of the talus and may reach the lateral talar tubercle, trigonal process, or os trigonum by expansion. Furthermore, the fibers can contribute to forming the tunnel of the flexor hallucis longus tendon. In the posterior view, the overall structure is triangular, with the vertex located laterally and the base situated medially (Fig. 8).

Another group of fibers originates at the upper edge of the ligament near its origin and courses in an upward, medial direction to the insertion site at the posterior edge of the tibia. These fibers fuse with the deep component of the posterior tibiofibular ligament (transverse ligament), reaching the posterior surface of the medial malleolus and helping to form the existing labrum in the posterior margin of the tibia. This group of fibers has been given several names

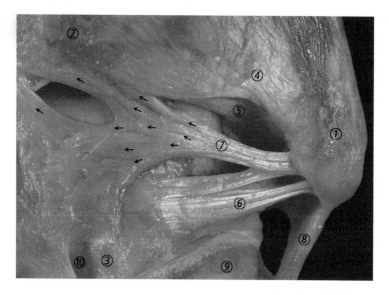

Fig. 8. Macrophotography of anatomic dissection of the posterior ligaments of the ankle. 1, lateral malleolus; 2, tibia; 3, talus (lateral talar process); 4, posterior tibiofibular ligament, superficial component; 5, transverse ligament or deep component of the posterior tibiofibular ligament; 6, posterior talofibular ligament; 7, posterior intermalleolar ligament (bundles indicated with arrows); 8, calcaneofibular ligament; 9, calcaneus; 10, tunnel for flexor hallucis longus tendon.

(capsular reinforcement bundle [38] or ascending or tibial bundle of the posterior talofibular ligament [6]), although the authors prefer the one proposed by Paturet [39]: posterior intermalleolar ligament. This ligament has been designated the "tibial slip" by Chen [40] and others [41] in several articles on arthroscopy (see Fig. 8; Fig. 9). The ligament is in close proximity to a synovial fold that runs transversally in a posterior recess of the ankle joint (Figs. 10 and 11) [40].

The posterior intermalleolar ligament has been the subject of recent studies because of its involvement in the posterior soft tissue impingement syndrome of the ankle [42,43]. Rosenberg and colleagues [44] observed this ligament in 56% of the dissections they performed and in 19% of patients in an MRI study, attributing the difference in frequency to the limited spatial resolution of MRI. In an MRI study of 23 classical ballet dancers who had symptoms of posterior

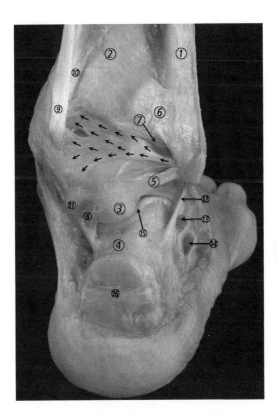

Fig. 9. Posterior view of anatomic dissection of the ankle ligaments. Posterior intermalleolar ligament and bundles indicated with arrows. 1, fibula; 2, tibia; 3, lateral talar process; 4, dorsal surface of the calcaneus; 5, posterior talofibular ligament; 6, superficial component of the posterior tibiofibular ligament; 7, transverse ligament or deep component of the posterior tibiofibular ligament; 8, flexor hallucis longus tendon with its retinaculum; 9, flexor digitorum longus tendon; 10, tibialis posterior tendon; 11, medial talar process; 12, calcaneofibular ligament; 13, peroneus brevis tendon; 14, peroneus longus tendon; 15, subtalar joint; 16, calcaneal tendon (cut at the level of insertion).

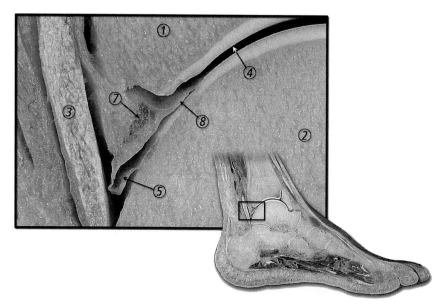

Fig. 10. Sagittal section of the ankle joint. Photomacrograph shows the relationship between the posterior intermalleolar ligament and the synovial fold. 1, tibia; 2, talus; 3, flexor hallucis longus tendon; 4, talocrural joint; 5, articular capsule (posterior recess); 6, posterior intermalleolar ligament; 7, synovial fold.

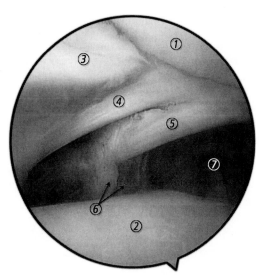

Fig. 11. Arthroscopic image of the posterior ligaments of the ankle through the anterior portal showing the constant relationship between the posterior intermalleolar ligament and the synovial fold. 1, plantar articular surface of the tibia; 2, dorsal articular surface of the talus; 3, synovial fringe; 4, transverse ligament or deep component of the posterior tibiofibular ligament; 5, posterior intermalleolar ligament; 6, synovial fold; 7, posterior articular capsule. (Courtesy of Prof. Pier Paolo Mariani, Department of Sports Traumatology, IUSM, University of Motor Sciences, Rome, Italy.)

ankle impingement syndrome, Peace and colleagues [45] detected the posterior intermalleolar ligament in 48% of the cases, a higher incidence than was found by Rosenberg and colleagues [44]. Peace and colleagues [45] ascribed the difference to the possibility that among these patients, the ligament would be more obvious on MRI because of scar thickening and inflammation resulting from repeated trauma. In their anatomic study, Milner and Soames [31] reported the presence of the posterior intermalleolar ligament in 72% of the specimens. Golanó and colleagues [27] identified this ligament in all of their dissections and in the arthroscopic study they performed. In the authors' opinion, the difference in frequency is probably due to the small size of the posterior intermalleolar ligament (mean, 2.3 mm; range, 1–5 mm) and the fact that it is difficult to dissect. In addition, the ligament may be divided into 2 or 3 different bands (20%) [44], of which none might not achieve bony insertion and become inserted in the joint capsule of the ankle (Fig. 9). After examination by arthroscopy, the division of this structure into bands should not be confused with an injury (Fig. 12).

In the posterior view, the posterior intermalleolar ligament is situated between the transverse ligament and the posterior talofibular ligament and runs obliquely from lateral to medial and from downward to upward (see Figs. 8 and 9). The posterior intermalleolar tenses during dorsiflexion and relaxes during plantar flexion [27]; therefore, trauma that causes forced dorsiflexion of the ankle can be assumed to produce injury to or rupture of this ligament or osteochondral avulsion [46]. Plantar flexion would cause it to relax and become susceptible to trapping between the tibia and the talus, leading to impingement. The possibility of impingement is accentuated by the presence of predisposing factors such as a trigonal process (Stieda process), an os trigonum, or a prominent dorsal process of the os calcis. The clinical relevance of the posterior intermalleolar ligament is manifested in the improvement of symptoms observed among patients treated with debridement of this ligament (Fig. 13) [27,42–44,47,48].

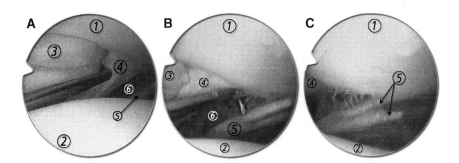

Fig. 12. (A–C) Arthroscopic images of the posterior ligaments of the ankle through the anteromedial portal showing the fascicles of the posterior intermalleolar ligament from lateral (A) to medial (C). 1, plantar articular surface of the tibia; 2, dorsal articular surface of the talus; 3, synovial fringe; 4, posterior tibiofibular ligament (deep component or transverse ligament); 5, posterior intermalleolar ligament; 6, gap between 4 and 5: intra-articular landmark to establish the posterolateral portal. (Courtesy of Dr. Raúl Puig-Adell, Barcelona, Spain.)

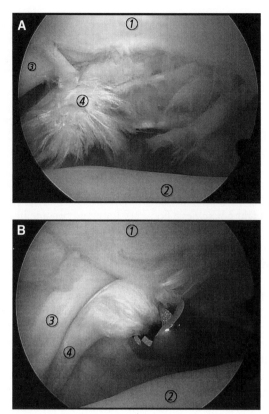

Fig. 13. (*A*) Arthroscopic view of posterior intermalleolar ligament rupture in a patient with posterior soft tissue impingement (right ankle). (*B*) Arthroscopic view of treatment. 1, plantar articular surface of the tibia; 2, dorsal articular surface of the talus; 3, transverse ligament or deep component of the posterior tibiofibular ligament; 4, posterior intermalleolar ligament. (Courtesy of Prof. Pier Paolo Mariani, Department of Sports Traumatology, IUSM, University of Motor Sciences, Rome, Italy.)

Van Dijk's [49] pioneer work on endoscopic portals has allowed observation of the posterior ligaments in ankle joint injuries. Palpation of these ligaments and neighboring structures has made it possible to identify and treat related pathology in the hindfoot. The use of these portals to treat posterior soft tissue impingement involving injury to the posterior intermalleolar ligament was recently described by Lohrer and Arentz [48].

Medial collateral ligament

The MCL is a strong, broad ligament with a multifascicular appearance that fans out from the medial malleolus toward the navicular, talus, and calcaneus. Because the origins and insertions of the various fascicles or components of the

MCL are contiguous and poorly defined, the anatomic descriptions show several interpretations, with artificial division being common. Most investigators appear to agree that the MCL has two layers: one superficial and one deep [14,50–52]. The ligaments that compose the superficial layer cross over two articulations (the ankle and the subtalar joints), whereas those composing the deep layer only cross the ankle joint [51]. Nevertheless, this differentiation is not entirely clear (Fig. 14) [50,53].

A review of the morphology of the medial malleolus is helpful to understand the origins of the MCL. In the medial view of the malleolus, two areas or segments (colliculi) can be seen, separated by the intercollicular groove, which is about 0.5 to 1 cm in length. The anterior segment or anterior colliculus is about 0.5 cm lower than the posterior segment or posterior colliculus [14]. The authors use this nomenclature because the international anatomic terminology [11] does not discuss these anatomic details and because it is used by most investigators in their anatomic descriptions.

The most commonly accepted description of the MCL is the one proposed by Milner and Soames [51] and later corroborated by Boss and Hintermann [50]. Six bands or components have been described for the MCL: three are always present (tibiospring ligament, tibionavicular ligament, and deep posterior

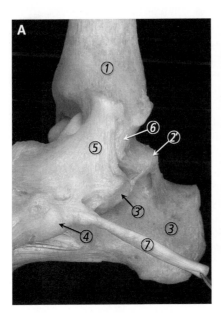
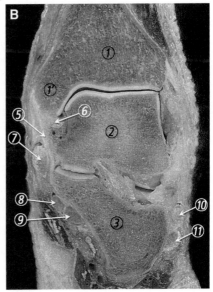

Fig. 14. (*A*) Medial view of the ankle joint ligaments showing their typical fanlike morphology. (*B*) Frontal section of the ankle joint where the superficial and deep layers of the MCL are separated by a small mass of fatty tissue. 1, tibia; 1′, medial malleolus; 2, talus; 2′, medial talar process; 3, calcaneus; 3′, sustentaculum tali; 4, navicular tuberosity; 5, superficial layer of the MCL; 6, deep layer of the MCL; 7, tibialis posterior tendon; 8, flexor digitorum longus tendon; 9, flexor hallucis longus tendon; 10, peroneus brevis tendon; 11, peroneus longus tendon.

tibiotalar ligament), whereas the presence of the other three may vary (superficial posterior tibiotalar ligament, tibiocalcaneal ligament, and deep anterior tibiotalar ligament) (Table 1).

Most of the MCL is covered by tendons as it extends down the leg to the bony insertions in the foot. The anterior region, in continuation with the joint capsule, is covered by the tendon of the posterior tibial muscle, and the middle and posterior area is covered by the tendons of the posterior tibial and long flexor muscles of the toes. The floor of the fibrosynovial sheaths covering these tendons is frequently composed of fibrocartilaginous tissue that is firmly adhered to the MCL. Precise dissection is needed to separate the fibrous sheath from the MCL. In the posterior region, the MCL continues with the posterior capsule of the ankle joint.

Although the description proposed by Milner and Soames [51] has been accepted, the anatomy of this ligament and its elements are still confusing. This confusion is partly because differentiation between the components during dissection is difficult and probably artificial because its origins and insertions are complex and because the nomenclature used still has not been reviewed and accepted by the Federative Committee on Anatomical Terminology [11]. Moreover, the images, sketches, and diagrams shown in the literature are imprecise [50].

Although injury to the MCL is far less common than LCL injury, it too can cause an impingement syndrome. According to the location of the fibrous tissue mass at the level of the medial recess and relative to the medial malleolus, the condition is differentiated into anteromedial soft tissue impingement, as described by Egol and Parisien [54], or posteromedial soft tissue impingement, as described by Liu and Mirzayan [55]. In any case, injury to the deep MCL is implicated in this kind of impingement. Anteromedial soft tissue impingement involves the anterior tibiotalar fascicle [56], whereas in posteromedial soft tissue impingement, the posterior tibiotalar ligament appears to be affected [57].

The mechanism of injury to this ligamentous complex is controversial: some investigators report that the most frequent mechanism is inversion [56,58], whereas others consider that eversion could also be a cause [55,59].

Table 1
Comparison of the nomenclature used for the medial collateral ligament components

Milner and Soames [31]	Sarrafian [14]
Superficial layer	
Tibiospring ligament (major component)	Tibioligamentous fascicle
Tibionavicular ligament (major component)	Tibionavicular fascicle and anterior superficial tibiotalar fascicle
Superficial tibiotalar ligament (additional band)	Superficial posterior tibiotalar ligament
Tibiocalcaneal ligament (additional band)	Tibiocalcaneal ligament
Deep layer	
Deep posterior tibiotalar ligament (major component)	Deep posterior tibiotalar ligament
Anterior deep tibiotalar ligament (additional band)	Deep anterior tibiotalar ligament

Summary

Following an ankle sprain, 10% to 50% of patients suffer some kind of chronic pain, usually caused by soft tissue impingement syndrome. Adequate knowledge of the anatomy of the ankle ligaments and the potential mechanisms for injury is key to understanding the role of these ligaments in the etiopathogenesis of soft tissue impingement syndrome.

Impingement syndromes of the ankle are usually caused by a sprain of some importance that has been treated improperly or inadequately because the patient wants to return to sports activity as soon as possible. The initial mechanism of injury determines the type of lesion sustained by the capsular and ligamentous structures, which can potentially progress to soft tissue impingement.

The mechanism of foot inversion is present in most ankle injuries and is the potential cause of impingement in any area. An inversion sprain can result in injury to the capsule, the LCL, the MCL, or the tibiofibular ligaments. The added influence of plantar flexion or dorsiflexion on the injury mechanism means that the lesion is predominantly anterior or posterior, respectively, and could lead to injury to other structures such as the posterior intermalleolar ligament, the osteochondral region of the neck of the talus, or the anteroinferior margin of the tibia.

The mechanism of foot eversion is more closely associated with injury to the medial capsular and ligamentous elements, although this is not the rule because an inversion sprain can also produce a lesion to these structures. Therefore, medial injury is probably more influenced by the rotating component of the subtalar joint to which the capsule and the MCL are subject.

Soft tissue impingement should be suspected in any case of chronic ankle pain secondary to a sprain. Although most sprains are usually due to inversion and lead to injury of lateral structures, the possibility of lesion to other regions should be considered.

Injury to the ligamentous and capsular structures induces the formation of scar and inflammatory tissue, leading to impingement. Surgical resection of this pathologic soft tissue has proved to be effective from subjective and objective viewpoints.

Acknowledgments

The authors thank Helen Casas and Celine Cavallo for the English translation of the text.

References

[1] Ferkel RD. Soft-tissue lesions of the ankle. In: Whipple TL, editor. Arthroscopic surgery: the foot and ankle. Philadelphia: Lippincott-Raven; 1996. p. 121–43.

[2] Renstrom FH, Lynch SA. Acute injuries of the ankle. Foot Ankle Clin 1999;4:697–711.

[3] Balduini FC, Tetzlaff J. Historical perspectives on injuries of the ligaments of the ankle. Clin Sports Med 1982;1:3–12.

[4] Anderson KJ, Lecoq JF. Operative treatment of injury to the fibular collateral ligament of the ankle. J Bone Joint Surg Am 1954;36:825–32.

[5] Clanton TO, Paul P. Syndesmosis injuries in athletes. Foot Ankle Clin N Am 2002;7:529–49.

[6] Testut L, Latarjet A. Tratado de anatomía humana [A treatise on human anatomy]. Barcelona, Spain: Salvat Editores, SA; 1985 [in Spanish].

[7] Morgan CD. Gross and arthroscopic anatomy of the ankle. In: McGuinty J, editor. Operative arthroscopy. Philadelphia: Lippincott-Raven; 1996. p. 1001–117.

[8] Ferkel RD, Scranton PE. Current concepts review: arthroscopy of the ankle and foot. J Bone Joint Surg Am 1993;75:1233–45.

[9] Shaffler GJ, Tirman PFJ, Stoller DW, et al. Impingement syndrome of the ankle following supination external rotation trauma: MR imaging findings with arthroscopic correlation. Eur Radiol 2003;13:1357–62.

[10] Kapanji IA. Cuadernos de fisiología articular [Joint physiology]. Cuaderno III. Barcelona, Spain: Masson, SA; 1982 [in Spanish].

[11] Federative Committee on Anatomical Terminology. Terminologia anatomica [Anatomical terminology]. Stuttgart, Germany: Thieme; 1998.

[12] Bartonícek J. Anatomy of the tibiofibular syndesmosis and its clinical relevance. Surg Radiol Anat 2003;25:379–86.

[13] Kelikian AS, Rinella AS. Ankle fractures. In: Kelikian AS, editor. Operative treatment of the foot and ankle. Stamford (CT): Appleton & Lange; 1999. p. 255–83.

[14] Sarrafian SK. Anatomy of the foot and ankle. Descriptive, topographic, functional. 2nd edition. Philadelphia: J.B. Lippincott Co.; 1993.

[15] Bassett III FH, Gates HS, Billys JB, et al. Talar impingement by the anteroinferior tibiofibular ligament. A cause of chronic pain in the ankle after inversion sprain. J Bone Joint Surg Am 1990;72:55–9.

[16] Akseki D, Pinar H, Bozkurt M, et al. The distal fascicle of the anterior inferior tibiofibular ligament as a cause of anterolateral ankle impingement. Results of arthroscopic resection. Acta Orthop Scand 1999;70:478–82.

[17] Nikolopoulos CE. Anterolateral instability of the ankle joint. An anatomical, experimental and clinical study [dissertation]. Athens, Greece: University of Athens; 1982.

[18] Nikolopoulus CE, Tsirikos AI, Sourmelis S, et al. The accessory anteroinferior tibiofibular ligament as a cause of talar impingement. A cadaveric study. J Sports Med 2004;32:389–95.

[19] Rasmussen O, Tovborg-Jensen I, Boe S. Distal tibiofibular ligaments, analysis of function. Acta Orthop Scand 1982;53:681–6.

[20] Johnson EE, Markolf KL. The contribution of the anterior talofibular ligament to ankle laxity. J Bone Joint Surg Am 1983;65:81–8.

[21] Akseki D, Pinar H, Yaldiz K, et al. The anterior inferior tibiofibular ligament and talar impingement: a cadaveric study. Knee Surg Sports Traumatol Arthrosc 2002;10:321–6.

[22] Ray RG, Kriz BM. Anterior inferior tibiofibular ligament. Variations and relationship to the talus. J Am Podiatr Med Assoc 1991;81:479–85.

[23] Liu SH, Raskin A, Osti L, et al. Arthroscopic treatment of anterolateral ankle impingement. Arthroscopy 1994;10:215–8.

[24] Horner G, Liu S. Arthroscopic treatment of talar impingement by the accessory anteroinferior tibiofibular ligament [abstract]. Arthroscopy 1996;12:384.

[25] Ferkel RD. Differential diagnosis of the chronic ankle sprain pain in the athlete. Sports Med Arthrosc Rev 1994;2:274–83.

[26] Kim S-H, Ha K-I. Arthroscopic treatment for impingement of the anterolateral soft tissues of the ankle. J Bone Joint Surg Br 2000;82:1019–21.

[27] Golanó P, Mariani PP, Rodríguez-Niedenfuhr M, et al. Arthroscopic anatomy of the posterior ankle ligaments. Arthroscopy 2002;18:353–8.

[28] Taylor DC, Englehardt DL, Bassett FH. Syndesmosis sprains of the ankle. The influence of heterotopic ossification. Am J Sport Med 1992;20:146–50.

[29] Milner CE, Soames RW. Anatomical variations of the anterior talofibular ligament of the human ankle joint [correspondence]. J Anat 1997;191:457–8.

[30] Burks RT, Morgan J. Anatomy of the lateral ankle ligaments. Am J Sport Med 1994;22:72–7.

[31] Milner CE, Soames RW. Anatomy of the collateral ligaments of the human ankle joint. Foot Ankle 1998;19:757–60.

[32] Delfaut EM, Demondion X, Boutry N, et al. Multi-fasciculated anterior talo-fibular ligament: reassessment of normal findings. Eur Radiol 2003;13:1836–42.

[33] Ferkel RD, Fisher SP. Progress in ankle arthroscopy. Clin Orthop 1989;240:210–20.

[34] Ferkel RD, Karzel RP, Del Pizzo W, et al. Arthroscopic treatment of anterolateral impingement of the ankle. Am J Sports Med 1991;19:440–6.

[35] Wolin I, Glassman F, Siderman S. Internal derangement of the talofibular component of the ankle. Surg Gynecol Obstet 1950;91:193–200.

[36] Trouilloud P, Dia A, Grammont P, et al. Variations du ligament calcaneo-fibulaire (lig. calcaneofibulare). Aplications à la cinématique de la cheville [Variations in the calcaneofibular ligament. Applications to ankle kinetics]. Bull Assoc Anat (Nancy) 1988;72:31–5 [in French].

[37] Ruth CJ. The surgical treatment of injuries of the fibular collateral ligaments of the ankle. J Bone Joint Surg Am 1961;43:233–6.

[38] Rouvière H, Delmas A. Anatomía Humana descriptiva, topográfica y funcional. Tomo III [Descriptive, topographic and functional human anatomy. Volume III]. 10th edition. Barcelona, Spain: Masson, SA; 1999 [in Spanish].

[39] Paturet G. Traité d'anatomie humaine [A treatise on human anatomy]. París: Masson; 1951 [in French].

[40] Chen Y. Arthroscopy of the ankle joint. In: Watanabe M, editor. Arthroscopy of small joints. New York: Igaku-Shoin; 1985. p. 104–27.

[41] Guhl JF. Soft tissue (synovial) pathology. In: Guhl JF, editor. Ankle arthroscopy. Thorofare (NJ): Slack, Inc.; 1988. p. 79–94.

[42] Hamilton WC. Foot and ankle injuries in dancers. Clin Sports Med 1988;7:143–73.

[43] Hamilton WG, Gepper MJ, Thompson FM. Pain in the posterior aspect of the ankle in dancers. Differential diagnosis and operative treatment. J Bone Joint Surg Am 1996;78:1491–500.

[44] Rosenberg ZS, Cheung YY, Beltran J, et al. Posterior intermalleolar ligament of the ankle: normal anatomy and MR imaging features. AJR Am J Roentgenol 1995;165:387–90.

[45] Peace KAL, Hillier JC, Hulme A, et al. MRI features of posterior ankle impingement syndrome in ballet dances: a review of 25 cases. Clin Radiol 2004;59:1025–33.

[46] Loren GJ, Ferkel RD. Arthroscopic strategies in fracture management of the ankle. In: Chow JCY, editor. Advanced arthroscopy. New York: Springer; 1999. p. 635–53.

[47] Fiorella D, Helms CA, Nunley II JA. The MR imaging features of the posterior intermalleolar ligament in patients with posterior impingement syndrome of the ankle. Skeletal Radiol 1999;28:573–6.

[48] Lohrer H, Arentz S. Posterior approach for arthroscopic treatment of posterolateral impingement syndrome of the ankle in a top-level field hockey player. Arthroscopy 2004;20:e15–21.

[49] van Dijk CN, Scholten PE, Krips R. A 2-portal endoscopic approach for diagnosis and treatment of posterior ankle pathology. Technical note. Arthroscopy 2000;16:871–6.

[50] Boss AP, Hintermann B. Anatomical study of the medial ankle ligament complex. Foot Ankle Int 2002;23:547–53.

[51] Milner CE, Soames RW. The medial collateral ligaments of the human ankle joint: anatomical variations. Foot Ankle 1998;19:289–92.

[52] Pankovich AM, Shivaram MS. Anatomical basis of variability in injuries of the medial malleolus and the deltoid ligament. I. Anatomical studies. Acta Orthop Scand 1979;50:217–23.

[53] Hintermann B. Medial ankle instability. Foot Ankle Clin N Am 2003;8:723–38.

[54] Egol KA, Parisien JS. Impingement syndrome of the ankle caused by a medial meniscoid lesion. Arthroscopy 1997;13:522–5.

[55] Liu SH, Mirzayan R. Posteromedial ankle impingement. Case report. Arthroscopy 1993;9: 709–11.

[56] Mosier-LaClair S, Monroe MT, Manoli A. Medial impingement syndrome of the anterior tibiotalar fascicle of deltoid ligament of the talus. Foot Ankle Int 2000;21:385–91.

[57] Koulouris G, Connell D, Schneider T, et al. Posterior tibiotalar ligament injury resulting in posteromedial impingement. Foot Ankle Int 2003;24:575–83.

[58] Paterson RS, Brown JN, Roberts SNJ. The posteromedial impingement lesion of the ankle. A series of six cases. Am J Sports Med 2001;29:550–7.

[59] Harper MC. Deltoid ligament: an anatomical evaluation of function. Foot Ankle 1987;8:19–22.

ELSEVIER
SAUNDERS

Foot Ankle Clin N Am
11 (2006) 297–310

FOOT AND
ANKLE CLINICS

Anterior Ankle Impingement

Johannes L. Tol, MD, PhD[a],*, C. Niek van Dijk, MD, PhD[b]

[a]*Department of Sports Medicine, Medical Center Haaglanden, P.O. Box 411,
2260 AK Leidschendam, The Netherlands*
[b]*Department of Orthopaedic Surgery, Academic Medical Center, P.O. Box 22660 1105 DD,
Amsterdam, The Netherlands*

Chronic ankle pain in athletes is caused commonly by formation of talotibial osteophytes at the anterior part of the ankle joint [1]. Morris [2] and later McMurray [3], named the condition "athlete's" ankle or "footballer's" ankle and described the treatment. McMurray stated that this injury is peculiar to the professional soccer player, especially those over the age of 25 years who have played for many years. In subsequent studies, this entity was described in other athletes, such as runners, ballet dancers, high jumpers, and volleyball players. The term "footballer's ankle" has been replaced by the anterior ankle impingement syndrome, and differentiation has been made between soft tissue impingement and bony impingement lesions [1,4,5].

Composition and etiology of osteophytes

Osteophytes are neoplastic cartilaginous and osseous protrusions around the joint space. Typically, they consist of five types of tissues: a superficial layer of mesenchymal fibrous connective tissue; fibrocartilage; hyaline cartilage; and deeper layers of hypertrophic cartilage and bone. The deeper layers become hypertrophic, vascularize, and undergo endochondral ossification [6]. Little is known about the exact cellular development and patterns of osteophytic formation. In osteoarthritis it is believed to be due to stimulation of cells at the chondrosynovial junction by polysaccharides that are derived from degradation of articular cartilage [7]; however, osteophytic formation also may occur without

---

* Corresponding author.
E-mail address: h.tol@mchaaglanden.nl (J.L. Tol).

weight-bearing articular cartilage damage, as seen in the bony impingement lesions [8].

Mechanical factors are believed to play an essential role in osteophytic formation. Several investigators tried to describe mechanical factors that could be influential. McMurray [3] attributed the development of the talotibial osteophytes to repeated capsule–ligamentar traction of the anterior ankle joint by repetitive kicking with the foot in full plantarflexion (eg, traction spurs). Since then, traction to the anterior ankle capsule during plantarflexion movements was supposed to be an important etiologic factor in the formation of anterior tibiotalar in the anterior ankle impingement syndrome (eg, traction spurs) [1,3,4,9,10]. This hypothesis is supported by the fact that these spurs are found frequently in athletes, who repetitively force their ankle in hyperplantarflexion actions that result in repetitive traction to the anterior joint capsule [11]. It assumes that the capsular attachment is located at the anterior cartilage rim, where the spurs originate.

A recent study, however, demonstrated that the anterior joint capsule attaches onto the tibia at an average of 6 mm proximal to the anterior cartilage rim [12]. On the talar side, the capsule attaches approximately 3 mm from the distal cartilage border. Therefore, the distance of capsule attachment from the site where bony spurs originate is large. Based on these anatomic observations, the hypothesis that talotibial spurs form as the result of recurrent traction to the joint capsule (traction spurs) is not plausible. This is supported by observations during arthroscopic surgery [13]. In patients who have bony impingement, the location of tibial spurs is at the joint level and within the confines of the joint capsule [13,14]. On the talar side, the typical osteophytes are found proximal to the talar neck notch. Tibial and talar osteophytes can be detected easily during an arthroscopic procedure with the ankle in forced dorsiflexion. The capsule does not have to be detached to locate these osteophytes.

O'Donoghue [15] considered the osteophytes to be related to direct mechanical trauma associated with the impingement of the anterior articular border of the tibia in the talar neck during forced dorsiflexion of the ankle joint. Here, bone formation is considered to be a response of the skeletal system to intermittent stress and injury, as evidenced by Wolff's law of bone remodeling [7]. According to Hawkins [16], runners, dancers, and high jumpers are prime examples of athletes who may be predisposed to this type of sports-related repeated trauma. Although this etiologic factor is cited widely [4,5,10,16], experimental support for both is scarce.

Along the distal tibia, the width of the nonweight bearing cartilage rim extends up to 3 mm proximal to the joint line. This nonweight bearing anterior cartilage rim undergoes the osteophytic transformation [5,12]. Damage to this anterior cartilage rim is known to occur in most supination traumas [17,18]. It was postulated that depending on the degree of damage, chondral and bone cell stimuli initiate a repair reaction with cartilage proliferation, scar tissue formation, and calcification. Additional damage by ankle sprains that are due to recurrent instability or forced dorsiflexion movements enhance this process [1]. Recent studies showed that chronic ankle instability is correlated significantly with os-teophytic formation in the medial ankle compartment [18,19]. Another factor in the development of spurs is recurrent microtrauma. It was demonstrated that spur formation in soccer players is related to recurrent ball impact, which can be regarded as repetitive microtrauma to the anteromedial aspect of the ankle [20]. Repetitive trauma to the anteromedial cartilage probably can be precluded by prevention of recurrent ankle sprains.

In the anterior ankle impingement syndrome the cause of pain is hypothesized not to be the osteophyte itself, but the inflamed soft tissue impingement that occurs between the osteophytes [14]. The tibial and talar spurs typically do not overlap each other [21]. Histopathologic analysis of arthroscopic resected soft tissue revealed synovial changes of chronic inflammation [22]. In cadaver specimens, a triangular soft tissue synovial fold, subsynovial fat, and collagen tissue were found along the entire anterior tibiotalar joint line. This soft tissue component gets squeezed between the anterior distal tibia and the talus during forced dorsiflexion movements. Recurrent trauma to this soft tissue component may lead to hypertrophy of the synovial layer, subsynovial fibrotic tissue for-mation, and infiltration of inflammatory cells. In theory, arthroscopic excision of the soft tissue could relieve pain. Talar and tibial osteophytes, however, de-crease the anterior space, and compression of this soft tissue component is more likely to occur. Therefore, in cases of bony anterior impingement lesions the authors believe that it is important to remove the osteophytes to restore the anterior space and to reduce the chance of symptoms recurring.

Clinical features

The typical patient is a young athlete with a history of recurrent inversion sprains [23]. The patient presents with vague, chronic anterior ankle pain; swelling after activity; and limited dorsiflexion [4]. Because of the complaints the patient often has had to reduce his (sporting) activities. McMurray [3] stated that the patient is able to kick the ball as well as ever when using the point of the toe, but feels a sudden stab of pain in front of the joint when attempting to kick it in the correct manner.

On physical examination there is recognizable local pain on palpation, which is present anteriorly. The osteophytes may be palpable with the ankle in slight plantarflexion.

A differentiation can be made between anteromedial and anterolateral im-pingement (Fig. 1). On palpation of the anterior joint line, the patient is asked if the test recreates his pain. Because the middle section (section II in Fig. 1) is covered by neurovascular structures and tendons, this part of the joint is diffi-cult to access by palpation. If a patient who has a clinical anterior impinge-ment syndrome experiences pain predominantly in section I when palpated, the diagnosis is anteromedial impingement. If pain on palpation is predominantly located in section III, the diagnosis is anterolateral impingement. Forced

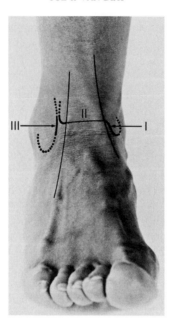

Fig. 1. Clinical differentiation between anteromedial and anterolateral impingement. At the anterior joint line the tibialis anterior muscle and the extensor digitorum longus muscle divide the anterior ankle joint in a medial section (section I), a middle section (section II), and lateral section (section III). (*From* Tol JL, Slim E, van Soest AJ, et al. The relationship of the kicking action in soccer and anterior ankle impingement syndrome. A biomechanical analysis. Am J Sports Med 2002;30(1): 45–50; with permission.)

hyperdorsiflexion can provoke the pain, but this movement often is not positive when examining the patient.

Radiographic features

The signs on standard lateral and anteroposterior radiographs vary according to the duration of symptoms. In the early stages there is slight periosteal roughening on the anterior aspect of the lower end of the tibia. Later, a bony ridge may be seen extending forward from the surface of the tibia. Occasionally, a similar bony outgrowth is seen projecting upward and slightly backward from the neck of the talus. The radiographic appearances are suggestive of osteoarthritis of the ankle joint with lipping of the articular margin of the tibia; however, there is no involvement of the articular surfaces, and the outgrowth lies slightly above the articular margin which often is unaffected [3].

Because of the anteromedial notch [24], anteromedial osteophytes are undetected on standard radiographs in a substantial number of patients who have anterior impingement complaints [25]. In a cadaver study, anteromedial tibial osteophytes that were up to 7.3 mm in size and originated from the anteromedial

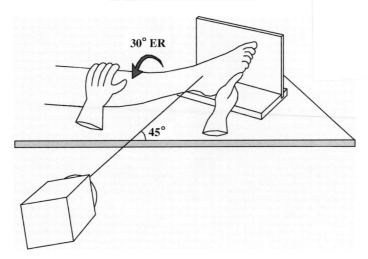

Fig. 2. 45/30 AMI ankle view: position of the foot relative to the x-ray beam. Starting from a standard lateral view, the x-ray beam is tilted into a 45° craniocaudal position with the lower extremity externally rotated (ER) 30°. The patient is asked to place his foot in the maximal plantarflexed position. The heel is placed on a 2-cm high shelf. The camera is rotated 10°, parallel to the anterior contour of the foot/ankle. The x-ray beam is centered just anterior to the lateral malleolus. A high-contrast mammography film (one-sided emulsion film) is used. This film is underexposed to 50% of the normal value for a standard ankle radiograph. (*From* van Dijk CN, et al. Oblique radiograph for the detection of bone spurs in anterior ankle impingement. Skeletal Radiol 2002;31(4):214–21; With kind permission of Springer Science and Business Media.)

border were undetected on a standard lateral radiograph because of superposition or overprojection of the more prominent anterolateral border of the distal tibia [25]. Medially located talar osteophytes remain undetected because of over-projection or superposition of the lateral part of the talar neck and body [25]. In these patients who have clinical symptoms of anterior ankle impingement, the diagnosis of soft tissue impingement is made, despite the fact that anteromedial osteophytes, ossicles, or posttraumatic calcification may be present [25].

Detection of the osteophytes is important for preoperative planning. Several investigators stated that surgical distinction between bony and soft tissue normal variants and pathologic conditions is difficult because of subtle variations in joint anatomy [24,26,27]. Especially in patients with accompanying synovial reflections that overlie the concealed osteophytes [24], anteromedial bony spurs are visualized poorly arthroscopically and can be missed. Radiographic classification of spur formation correlates with the outcome of surgery [5,8,13]. An oblique radiograph was introduced to detect medially located tibial and talar osteophytes. In this oblique anteromedial impingement (AMI) view, the beam is tilted in a 45° craniocaudal direction with the leg in 30° of external rotation and the foot in plantarflexion (Fig. 2).

The sensitivity of lateral radiographs for detecting anterior tibial and talar osteophytes was 40% and 32%, respectively (specificity 70% and 82%) [28]. When the lateral radiograph was combined with an oblique AMI radiograph, the

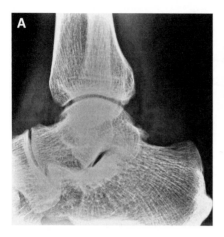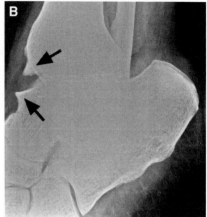

Fig. 3. Anteromedial ankle pain in a 39-year-old man. At age 21 years he sustained a lateral ankle ligament rupture. Progressive anteromedial pain with intermittent swelling and 5° of limited dorsiflexion (compared with the uninvolved ankle) developed after a new inversion trauma at age 37 years. (*A*) The standard anteroposterior and lateral views do not show any abnormality. (*B*) On the AMI view, bony spurs are visible on the anteromedial tibial rim (*upper arrow*) and on the talar neck (*lower arrow*). Both osteophytes were confirmed and removed successfully during arthroscopic surgery. (*From* van Dijk CN, et al. Oblique radiograph for the detection of bone spurs in anterior ankle impingement. Skeletal Radiol 2002;31(4):214–21; With kind permission of Springer Science and Business Media.)

sensitivities increased to 85% and 73%, respectively. This increase was due to the high sensitivity of the oblique AMI radiographs for detecting anteromedial osteophytes (93% for tibial and 67% for talar osteophytes). A lateral radiograph is insufficient to detect all anteriorly located osteophytes; an oblique AMI radiograph is a useful adjunct to routine radiographs and is recommended to detect anteromedial tibial and talar osteophytes (Figs. 3 and 4).

Treatment and outcome

Conservative treatment, consisting of intra-articular injections or heel lifts, is recommended in the early stages; however, frequently it is unsuccessful [4,9]. McMurray [3] reported the first patients who were treated surgically. After the removal of anteriorly located osteophytes by open arthrotomy the patients successfully returned to professional soccer. In subsequent studies, numerous investigators reported good results with open arthrotomy [15,29,30]. Open arthrotomy can be complicated by cutaneous nerve entrapment, damage of the long extensor tendons, wound dehiscence, and formation of hypertrophic scar tissue [4].

Before the advent of arthroscopy of the ankle joint, it was believed that this technique was unsuitable in view of the narrow joint space and convex talar anatomy. The first arthroscopic inspection of cadaver ankle joints was performed by Burman [31] in 1931. It is used widely today.

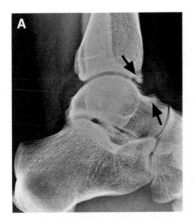
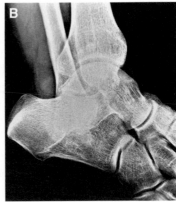

Fig. 4. A 52-year-old patient sustained a pronation trauma of the right ankle 7 months before visiting the orthopedic department with anterior ankle pain. Dorsiflexion was 10° compared with 15° in the left ankle. The lateral radiograph (*A*) shows an osteophyte which is not visible on the AMI view (*B*), which indicates that the osteophyte is located laterally. The lateral location was confirmed during arthroscopy. (*From* van Dijk CN, et al. Oblique radiograph for the detection of bone spurs in anterior ankle impingement. Skeletal Radiol 2002;31(4):214–21; With kind permission of Springer Science and Business Media.)

During arthroscopy the patient is placed in a supine position with slight elevation of the ipsilateral buttock. The heel of the affected foot rests on the end of the operating table, which makes it possible for the surgeon to dorsiflex the ankle joint fully by leaning against the sole of the patient's foot (Fig. 5). After making an anteromedial skin incision, the subcutaneous layer is divided bluntly with a hemostat. A 4-mm, 30°-angle arthroscope is used routinely. The anterolateral portal is made under arthroscopic control. Additional portals, just anterior to the tip of the lateral or medial malleolus portal, are used only when indicated.

Osteophytes are removed using a 4-mm chisel and motorized shaver system (bone cutter or small acromionizer). These spurs can be identified easily when the ankle is in a fully dorsiflexed position (Fig. 5). The authors do not use distraction of the joint because it results in tightening of the anterior capsule, which makes it more difficult to identify the osteophytes. Another advantage of the forced dorsiflexion position is that the talus is concealed in the joint, which protects the weight-bearing cartilage of the talus from potential iatrogenic damage (see Fig. 5). The contour of the anterior tibia is identified by shaving away the tissue just superior to the osteophyte (see Fig. 4A). In case of osteophytes or ossicles at the tip of the medial malleolus an overcorrection of the medial malleolus generally is performed by shaving some of it away after resection of the osteophyte (see Fig. 4B).

Postoperative rehabilitation treatment consists of a compression bandage and partial weight bearing for 3 to 5 days. The patient is instructed to dorsiflex the ankle and foot actively upon awakening and to repeat this exercise a few times every hour for the first 2 to 3 days after surgery [13].

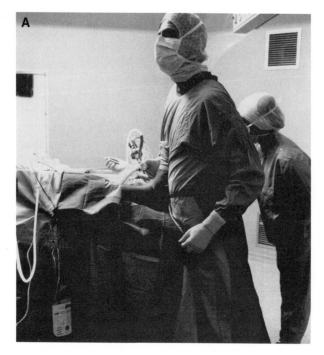

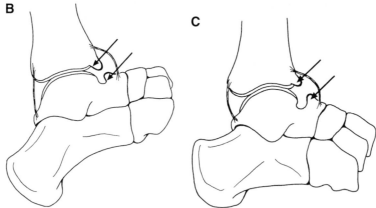

Fig. 5. Surgical procedure. (*A*) The heel rests on the end of the operating table, which makes it possible for the surgeon to dorsiflex the ankle joint fully by leaning against the sole of the patient's foot. (*B*) In the dorsiflexed position, filling the joint with saline causes the anterior compartment to "open up." All structures in front of the medial malleolus, the lateral malleolus, and the front of the distal tibia and talar neck can be inspected and treated easily. The arrows point to the osteophytes on the distal tibia and talar neck. (*C*) Distraction of the joint results in tightening of the anterior joint capsule, which makes it more difficult to identify the structures in the anterior compartment. The arrows point to the osteophytes on the distal tibia and talar neck. (*From* van Dijk CN, Tol JL, Verheyen CC. A prospective study of prognostic factors concerning the outcome of arthroscopic surgery for anterior ankle impingement. Am J Sports Med 1997;25(6):737–45; with permission.)

In the late 1980s, several investigators presented (retrospective) studies of treatment of the anterior ankle impingement syndrome. Hawkins [16] reported on three case studies of athletes who were treated successfully with an average follow-up of 3 years. In 1989, Martin and colleagues [32] presented the retrospective results of 57 patients who were treated arthroscopically (Fig. 6). Of these 57 patients, 7 patients had anteriorly located osteophytes; six of the seven ankles had anterior synovitis in addition to the osteophytes. Based on a seven-grade subjective and functional scoring system, 57% had good or excellent results. The overall complication rate, including infections, paresthesias, and hemarthrosis,

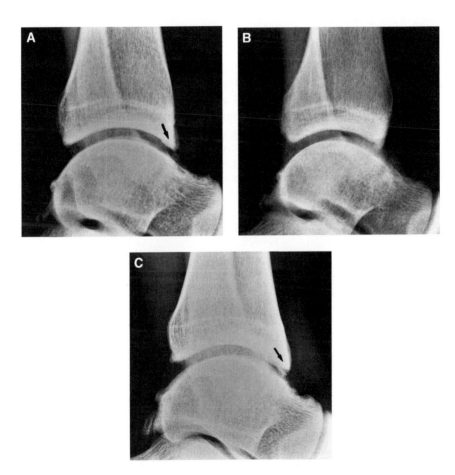

Fig. 6. Lateral radiographs of the ankle of a 25-year-old man who had a grade I lesion. (*A*) The preoperative radiograph shows an osteophyte (*arrow*) that was removed arthroscopically. (*B*) After removal of the osteophyte the anterior tibial contour is normal. (*C*) At 5.5 years of follow-up the osteophyte has recurred (*arrow*). The scores for patient satisfaction and successful treatment were good. (*From* Tol JL, Verheyen CP, van Dijk CN. Arthroscopic treatment of anterior impingement in the ankle. J Bone Joint Surg Br 2001;83(1):9–13; with permission, © 2001 British Editorial Society of Bone and Joint Surgery.)

was 15%. Application of a comparable scoring system showed that 87% of patients had good/excellent results in a retrospective series of 30 cases at an average of 2 years of follow-up. For synovitis (12 cases), osteophytes and loose bodies (6 cases), and osteoarthritis (6 cases) the percentage of good/excellent results were 80%, 100%, and 0%, respectively. The complication rate was 10%.

A success rate of approximately 67% was reported in the first series of arthroscopically treated ankles from Biedert [1] and Feder and Schonholtz [33]. Ferkel and colleagues [22] reported on 31 patients who had soft tissue impingement lesions. Histopathologic analysis of the arthroscopically resected tissue revealed synovial changes with chronic inflammation. The success rate was 84%. Comparable high percentages of good/excellent results after arthroscopic treatment of synovial impingement lesions were reported by other investigators [5,34–36]. Less favorable results and a high percentage of (18%) temporary neurologic complications were reported in a series by Jerosch and colleagues [37]. Although there was a significant decrease in pain score, only 26% of the patients reached their previous level of athletic activity.

The first study with results of treatment of isolated anterior bony ankle impingement lesions was published by Ogilvie-Harris and colleagues [10]. Patients were rated pre- and postoperatively according to a five-grade scoring system; pain, swelling, stiffness, limping, and activity were recorded. At an average of 39 months of follow-up (range, 24–68 months), 15 of the 17 patients reported significant improvement. There were residual osteophytes in two ankles at follow-up review. The complication rate was 18% (one case of superficial infection and two cases of residual numbness).

In the Belgian literature, a series of 13 soccer players who were treated for bony impingement revealed 92% good/excellent results [38]. Amendola and colleagues [39] published the results of a prospective study of 79 consecutive ankle arthroscopies. Fifteen cases of soft tissue impingement lesions and 14 cases of anterior bony impingement lesions were included. At a minimum follow-up of 2 years (range, 24–42 months) both groups showed a statistically significant decrease of subjective analog scores that included pain, swelling, and effectiveness of the ankle arthroscopy. Eighty percent of the soft tissue impingement lesions and 86% of the anterior bony impingement lesions benefited from the procedure. Three patients (complication rate, 18%) had neurologic complaints: two cases of partial deep peroneal nerve neurapraxia and one case of superficial peroneal nerve irritation.

Scranton and McDermott [8] published the only study that compared open and arthroscopic resection of the impinging osteophytes. The patients who were treated arthroscopically recovered in approximately half the time, and returned to full athletic training 1 month faster. They also showed that the radiological size and location of the osteophytes correlated with the outcome of surgery. Although the investigators mentioned that no effort was made to select patients for one form of treatment or the other, it is questionable whether the two groups were comparable. They missed the unique chance to publish the only randomized clinical study to compare open versus arthroscopic treatment.

Table 1
Classification for osteoarthritic changes of the ankle joint

Grade	Characteristics
Grade 0	Normal joint or subchondral sclerosis
Grade I	Osteophytes without joint space narrowing
Grade II	Joint space narrowing with or without osteophytes
Grade III	(Sub)total disappearance/deformation of the joint space

In the authors' series [25], differentiation was made between patients who had osteophytes with and without joint space narrowing. There is a significant difference in prognosis between these two types of osteophytes. Osteophytes without joint space narrowing (grade 0/I) are not a manifestation of osteoarthritis, and subsequently, a "normal" joint remains after removal of these spurs. Because none of the existing scoring systems take this into account, the authors developed and used a classification for ankle osteoarthritic changes (Table 1). Patients who had osteophytes without joint space narrowing (grade I, 82% good/excellent results) showed significantly better results than did patients who had joint space narrowing (grade II, 50% good/excellent results; Table 2). In accordance with the literature, patients who had grade III osteoarthritis were considered to be unsuitable for arthroscopic debridement [1].

At 5 to 8 years of follow-up osteophytes recurred in two thirds of the ankles with grade I lesions. Coull and colleagues [40] reported recurrence of osteophytes in all 27 of their patients who underwent open debridement. All patients in whom osteophytes recurred had a history of ongoing supination trauma or repetitive forced dorsiflexion, most often as a result of regular participation in soccer. There was no statistical correlation between the recurrence of osteophytes and the return of symptoms. Cheng and Ferkel [41] found asymptomatic bony spurs in the ankles of 45% patients who played football and 59% of patients who were dancers. Asymptomatic ankles may become painful when anterior hypertrophic synovial or scar tissue impedes movement [1,8,9] after major surgery [42]. Usually, removal of the soft tissue relieves symptoms [1,8,13].

Table 2
Percentage excellent/good results for patient satisfaction and for a five-parameter scoring system for successful treatment in relation to the osteoarthritic classification in 57 patients 5 to 8 years after arthroscopic debridement of the ankle for anterior ankle impingement

		Excellent/good result (%)	
		Patient satisfaction	Successful treatment
Grade	N	Total	Total
0	10	100	100
I	30	77	73
II	17	53	29
Overall	57	74	65

There were accompanying soft tissue changes (synovitis or scar tissue) in all of the authors' patients who had anterior osteophytic impingement. It was a consistent finding at arthroscopy that the hypertrophic synovial tissue impinged between the osteophytes during forced dorsiflexion. At follow-up, most of the ankles in which osteophytes had recurred were asymptomatic. The osteophytes themselves are not painful; the compression of the synovial fold or fibrotic (scar) tissue causes pain. In theory, arthroscopic excision of the soft tissue can relieve pain. Talar and tibial osteophytes, however, reduce the anterior joint space. After arthroscopy, a postoperative hematoma may develop which again forms an anterior impediment. Therefore, it is important to restore the anterior space and reduce the chance of symptoms recurring.

There are few descriptions of arthroscopic management of the osteoarthritic ankle. Ogilvie-Harris and Sekyi-Otu [43] used a subjective and functional scoring system to define successful treatment. At a mean follow-up of 45 months, there were only a few excellent or good results; however, 63% of patients reported marked improvement and were satisfied with the procedure. These favorable results are supported by some investigators [41] and refuted by others [1,32,44]. Patient satisfaction was excellent or good in 53% of the authors' patients who had grade II osteoarthritic changes. Rated on the ankle scoring system, which includes objective parameters, such as swelling, only 29% of results were good or excellent; four patients had only poor or fair results, yet all expressed overall satisfaction. The lack of correlation between patient satisfaction and the scoring system [10] makes it difficult to evaluate a surgical procedure. Validated scoring systems are useful for comparing different clinical trials, but their objective criteria seem to be of little importance to the individual patient. Our results lend support to the view of Ogilvie-Harris and Sekyi-Otu that only subjective criteria should be used to evaluate outcomes [43].

In the authors' prospective series, with the exception of three patients who needed additional surgery, all patients who had grade II lesions (osteophytes with joint space narrowing) had less pain at follow-up. Approximately half of them rated their satisfaction as excellent or good. In most ankles, narrowing of the joint space had not progressed. Given that the alternative is arthrodesis, these results are acceptable. Nevertheless, patients should be informed of the limitations of the procedure and the possibility of reoperation.

Summary

Anterior ankle impingement syndrome is a pain syndrome that is characterized by anterior ankle pain on (hyper) dorsiflexion. On investigation there is recognizable pain on the anteromedial or anterolateral aspect of the ankle joint. Some swelling or limitation of dorsiflexion is present. A plain radiograph can reveal the cause of the impingement. Plain radiographs often are negative in patients who have AMI; an oblique view is recommended in these patients. Arthroscopic excision of soft tissue overgrowths and osteophytes is an effective way of treating anterior impingement of the ankle in patients who have no narrowing of the joint space. For grade II lesions (osteophytes secondary to arthritis with joint space narrowing) the long-term good/excellent result is still 50%. Arthroscopic treatment is still a good option in these patients; with the exception of an arthrodesis or a prothesis no other therapeutic option is available.

References

[1] Biedert R. Anterior ankle pain in sports medicine: aetiology and indications for arthroscopy. Arch Orthop Trauma Surg 1991;110(6):293–7.

[2] Morris LH. Report of cases of athlete's ankle. J Bone Joint Surg 1943;25:220.

[3] McMurray TP. Footballer's ankle. J Bone Joint Surg 1950;32:68–9.

[4] Cutsuries AM, Saltrick KR, Wagner J, et al. Arthroscopic arthroplasty of the ankle joint. Clin Podiatr Med Surg 1994;11(3):449–67.

[5] Ferkel RD, Fasulo GJ. Arthroscopic treatment of ankle injuries. Orthop Clin North Am 1994; 25(1):17–32.

[6] Aigner T, Dietz U, Stoss H, et al. Differential expression of collagen types I, II, III, and X in human osteophytes. Lab Invest 1995;73(2):236–43.

[7] Williams JM, Brandt KD. Exercise increases osteophyte formation and diminishes fibrillation following chemically induced articular cartilage injury. J Anat 1984;139(Pt 4):599–611.

[8] Scranton Jr PE, McDermott JE. Anterior tibiotalar spurs: a comparison of open versus arthroscopic debridement. Foot Ankle 1992;13(3):125–9.

[9] Ferkel RD, Scranton Jr PE. Arthroscopy of the ankle and foot. J Bone Joint Surg Am 1993; 75(8):1233–42.

[10] Ogilvie-Harris DJ, Mahomed N, Demaziere A. Anterior impingement of the ankle treated by arthroscopic removal of bony spurs. J Bone Joint Surg Br 1993;75(3):437–40.

[11] Handoll HH, Rowe BH, Quinn KM, et al. Interventions for preventing ankle ligament injuries. Cochrane Database Syst Rev 2001;3:CD000018.

[12] Tol JL, van Dijk CN. Etiology of the anterior ankle impingement syndrome: a descriptive anatomical study. Foot Ankle Int 2004;25(6):382–6.

[13] van Dijk CN, Tol JL, Verheyen CC. A prospective study of prognostic factors concerning the outcome of arthroscopic surgery for anterior ankle impingement. Am J Sports Med 1997;25(6): 737–45.

[14] Tol JL, Verheyen CP, van Dijk CN. Arthroscopic treatment of anterior impingement in the ankle. J Bone Joint Surg Br 2001;83(1):9–13.

[15] O'Donoghue DH. Impingement exostoses of the talus and the tibia. J Bone Joint Surg 1957;39: 835–52.

[16] Hawkins RB. Arthroscopic treatment of sports-related anterior osteophytes in the ankle. Foot Ankle 1988;9(2):87–90.

[17] van Dijk CN. On diagnostic strategies in patients with severe ankle sprain. [Thesis] University of Amsterdam.

[18] van Dijk CN, Bossuyt PM, Marti RK. Medial ankle pain after lateral ligament rupture. J Bone Joint Surg Br 1996;78(4):562–7.

[19] Krips R, Brandsson S, Swensson C, van Dijk CN, et al. Anatomical reconstruction and Evans tenodesis of the lateral ligaments of the ankle. Clinical and radiological findings after follow-up for 15 to 30 years. J Bone Joint Surg Br 2002;84(2):232–6.

[20] Tol JL, Slim E, van Soest AJ, et al. The relationship of the kicking action in soccer and anterior ankle impingement syndrome. A biomechanical analysis. Am J Sports Med 2002;30(1): 45–50.

[21] Berberian WS, Hecht PJ, Wapner KL, et al. Morphology of tibiotalar osteophytes in anterior ankle impingement. Foot Ankle Int 2001;22(4):313–7.

[22] Ferkel RD, Karzel RP, Del Pizzo W, et al. Arthroscopic treatment of anterolateral impingement of the ankle. Am J Sports Med 1991;19(5):440-6.

[23] St Pierre RK, Velazco A, Fleming LL. Impingement exostoses of the talus and fibula secondary to an inversion sprain. A case report. Foot Ankle 1983;3(5):282-5.

[24] Ray RG, Gusman DN, Christensen JC. Anatomical variation of the tibial plafond: the antero-medial tibial notch. J Foot Ankle Surg 1994;33(4):419-26.

[25] van Dijk CN, Wessel RN, Tol JL, et al. Oblique radiograph for the detection of bone spurs in anterior ankle impingement. Skeletal Radiol 2002;31(4):214-21.

[26] Ferkel RD. Arthroscopic surgery: the foot and the ankle. Philadelphia: Lippincott-Raven; 1996.

[27] Vogler HW, Stienstra JJ, Montgomery F, et al. Anterior ankle impingement arthropathy. The role of anterolateral arthrotomy and arthroscopy. Clin Podiatr Med Surg 1994;11(3):425-47.

[28] Tol JL, Verhagen RA, Krips R, et al. The anterior ankle impingement syndrome: diagnostic value of oblique radiographs. Foot Ankle Int 2004;25(2):63-8.

[29] Hensley JP, Saltrick K, Le T. Anterior ankle arthroplasty: a retrospective study. J Foot Surg 1990;29(2):169-72.

[30] Parkes II JC, Hamilton WG, Patterson AH, et al. The anterior impingement syndrome of the ankle. J Trauma 1980;20(10):895-8.

[31] Burman MS. Arthroscopy of direct visualization of joints. An experimental cadaver study. J Bone Joint Surg 1931;13:669-95.

[32] Martin DF, Baker CL, Curl WW, et al. Operative ankle arthroscopy. Long-term followup. Am J Sports Med 1989;17(1):16-23 [discussion 23].

[33] Feder KS, Schonholtz GJ. Ankle arthroscopy: review and long-term results. Foot Ankle 1992; 13(7):382-5.

[34] Clasper JC, Pailthorpe CA. Chronic ankle pain in soldiers: the role of ankle arthroscopy and soft tissue excision. J R Army Med Corps 1996;142(3):107-9.

[35] Meislin RJ, Rose DJ, Parisien JS, et al. Arthroscopic treatment of synovial impingement of the ankle. Am J Sports Med 1993;21(2):186-9.

[36] Thein R, Eichenblat M. Arthroscopic treatment of sports-related synovitis of the ankle. Am J Sports Med 1992;20(5):496-8.

[37] Jerosch J, Steinbeck J, Schroder M, Halm H. Arthroscopic treatment of anterior synovitis of the ankle in athletes. Knee Surg Sports Traumatol Arthrosc 1994;2(3):176-81.

[38] Reynaert P, Gelen G, Geens G. Arthroscopic treatment of anterior impingement of the ankle. Acta Orthop Belg 1994;60(4):384-8.

[39] Amendola A, Petrik J, Webster-Bogaert S. Ankle arthroscopy: outcome in 79 consecutive patients. Arthroscopy 1996;12(5):565-73.

[40] Coull R, Raffiq T, James LE, et al. Open treatment of anterior impingement of the ankle. J Bone Joint Surg Br 2003;85(4):550-3.

[41] Cheng JC, Ferkel RD. The role of arthroscopy in ankle and subtalar degenerative joint disease. Clin Orthop Relat Res 1998;(349):65-72.

[42] van Dijk CN, Verhagen RA, Tol JL. Arthroscopy for problems after ankle fracture. J Bone Joint Surg Br 1997;79(2):280-4.

[43] Ogilvie-Harris DJ, Sekyi-Otu A. Arthroscopic debridement for the osteoarthritic ankle. Arthroscopy 1995;11(4):433-6.

[44] Cerulli G, Caraffa A, Buompadre V, et al. Operative arthroscopy of the ankle. Arthroscopy 1992; 8(4):537-40.

ELSEVIER
SAUNDERS

Foot Ankle Clin N Am
11 (2006) 311–329

FOOT AND
ANKLE CLINICS

Ankle Instability

Rover Krips, MD, PhD*, Jasper de Vries, MD,
C. Niek van Dijk, MD, PhD

*Department of Orthopaedic Surgery, Academic Medical Center, P.O. Box 22700,
1100 DD Amsterdam, The Netherlands*

The ankle joint is the most congruent joint of the human body. Stability is provided by the bony configuration of the ankle mortise and the talar dome and by the ankle ligaments. During ankle motions, rotation and translation around and along the movement axes occur. Soft tissue stability is provided mainly by the ligaments; these are the tibio-fibular syndesmosis superiorly, the deltoid ligament on the medial and lateral sides, the anterior talo-fibular ligament, the calcaneo-fibular ligament, and the posterior talo-fibular ligament (Fig. 1) [1]. The anterior talo-fibular ligament can be considered to be an intra-articular reinforcement of the joint capsule. This ligament is the main stabilizer on the lateral aspect of the ankle and is the most vulnerable to injuries [2]. The anterior talo-fibular ligament is in a plane parallel to the axis of movement (flexion-extension), if the ankle is in a neutral position. Thus, the anterior talo-fibular ligament is a true collateral ligament when the foot is placed in plantar flexion. Most ankle ligament injuries occur by internal rotation in the equinus position with the foot in plantar flexion, when the narrowest part of the talus is placed in the ankle mortise and the ankle, is thus, rendered most lax. This is probably an important reason for the high prevalence of injuries of the anterior talo-fibular ligament [2–4].

The extra-articular calcaneo-fibular ligament arises from the anterior part of the tip of the fibula. It runs obliquely downward and backward to be attached to the lateral surface of the calcaneus. There is a great variety in direction and in proximal attachment. Usually, the main part attaches to the tip of the fibula, and in most cases, a bundle of fibers also runs directly to the anterior talo-fibular ligament. In some cases, the calcaneo-fibular ligament attaches predominantly to the anterior talo-fibular ligament [1,5]. In contrast to the anterior talo-fibular

---

* Corresponding author.
E-mail address: roverkrips@hotmail.com (R. Krips).

1083-7515/06/$ – see front matter © 2006 Elsevier Inc. All rights reserved.
doi:10.1016/j.fcl.2006.02.003

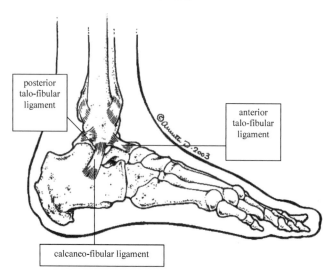

Fig. 1. The lateral ankle ligaments.

ligament, it is not part of the fibrous capsule but is separated from it. The calcaneofibular ligament is associated intimately with the posteromedial part of the peroneal tendon sheath, and bridges the talocrural and the subtalar joints. The posterior talo-fibular ligament is a short and thick ligament. It is tight with the ankle in extension and lax in plantar flexion. Injuries to this ligament are infrequent, and the ligament is not used as a part of a reconstructive procedure.

The distal tibiofibular syndesmosis is essential for stability of the ankle mortise, and thereby, to weight transmission and walking. Experimentally, a combination of forced external rotation, dorsiflexion, and axial loading of the ankle caused a rupture of the anterior tibio-fibular ligament [2,3]. This might be accompanied by a partial rupture of the deltoid ligament. The main stabilizer on the medial side is the deep portion of the deltoid ligament, which is fan-shaped, thick, and strong and is injured infrequently.

Anatomic variations in shape, size, orientation, and capsular relations of the lateral ankle ligaments are common; up to 75% of subjects show some variation, most commonly in the calcaneo-fibular ligament. The anterior talo-fibular ligament is divided into two separate bundles in one third of all patients [5]. These anatomic variations should be borne in mind when deciding upon treatment of ankle ligament injuries, especially when considering surgical reconstruction of the calcaneo-fibular ligament [6].

Acute ligament injuries

Acute ankle ligament injury is the single most common type of injury that is seen by general practitioners and emergency departments. They account for approximately 25% of all injuries of the musculoskeletal system; more than 20,000 patients are seen in the United States each day for this type of injury [5,7]. A rupture of the lateral ankle ligaments is present in approximately 10% to 15% of all inversion trauma [8].

In most cases the lateral ligament injury occurs with the foot rotating inward in plantar flexion when the tibia is rotating outward simultaneously; this gives rise to anterolateral rotational movement. The medial malleolus acts as a fulcrum when the ankle moves into increased inversion; it loses its stabilizing function and increases the strain on the lateral side.

Often, ankle ligament injuries are classified as grade I (mild), grade II (moderate), and grade III (severe) [9]. Grade I injuries include stretching of the ligament without macroscopic rupture. There is a minor swelling and tenderness but not an increased laxity. The loss of function is minimal and the recovery usually is quick. In grade II injuries there is a partial macroscopic rupture of the ligaments, with moderate swelling, tenderness, and pain. There is a mild to moderate increment of laxity, some loss of motion, and moderate functional disability.

Grade III injuries always include a complete rupture of the ligaments and the joint capsule, with severe bruising, swelling, and pain. There is a major loss of function, reduction of motion, and increased laxity due to the ligament rupture. The injured subject often is unable to bear weight because of pain. Radiographs are needed often to rule out a fracture. The value of this classification is doubtful, because a partial rupture or isolated capsular lesion (grade I) is present in less than 1% of cases. Several studies showed that there is no difference between the prognosis of a single (grade II) or a multiple ligament rupture (grade III) [5,10–12]. Therefore, after a supination trauma it is important to distinguish a simple sprain from a ligament rupture.

It has been shown that a rupture of the anterior talo-fibular ligament occurs as an isolated injury in 50% to 75% of cases. A partial rupture of this anterior talo-fibular ligament or an isolated capsular lesion is present in only 1% of patients after a supination injury [2,13]. With an increasing force, the calcaneo-fibular ligament also is ruptured. A rupture of the anterior talo-fibular ligament and the calcaneo-fibular ligament occurs in 15% to 25% of cases. Isolated rupture of the calcaneo-fibular ligament happens in approximately 1% of patients, and injury to the posterior talo-fibular ligament is extremely rare [2,14,15].

Isolated ligament injuries of the deltoid ligament are infrequent. The frequency has been estimated to be approximately 2.5% of all ankle ligament injuries [4]. The injury mechanism is an excessive eversion (ie, outward rotation of the foot during simultaneous inward rotation of the tibia). This type of injury usually takes several weeks to heal, and more often gives rise to chronic anteromedial pain rather than recurrent medial instability. Pain and swelling are present for a longer period of time than for a corresponding injury on the lateral side.

Injury of the ankle syndesmosis is seen often in soccer players after external rotation of the foot; in dancers after forced dorsiflexion of the foot; or in alpine skiers after combined external rotation, axial compression, and forced dorsiflexion [16–18]. When this injury is suspected, a complete radiographic examination of the lower leg should be performed to rule out a fracture of the proximal fibula. Disruption of the ankle syndesmosis is painful, and often heals slowly; however, residual disability with recurrent episodes of instability is not frequent [19,20]. Usually, a rupture of the anterior tibio-fibular ligament alone does not cause symptoms or degenerative changes at long-term follow-up. It is concluded that this rupture of the anterior tibio-fibular ligament does occur in 1% to 5% of patients after severe inversion trauma of the ankle [19,21]. Physical examination cannot discriminate between an isolated lateral ankle ligament rupture and a lateral ankle ligament rupture that is accompanied by a (partial) syndesmotic ligament rupture. Treatment of the lateral ankle ligament rupture is sufficient for the natural healing of the concomitant syndesmotic ligament rupture [18–20].

A supination trauma is associated with a distraction force on the lateral side and a compression force on the medial side of the joint [22]. Damage to the cartilage rim that covers the anterior distal tibia, the anterior part of the medial malleolus, and the medial talar facet is known to occur in most patients who sustain a supination trauma. Depending on the degree of damage, a repair reaction with cartilage proliferation, scar tissue formation, calcification, and eventually, development of osteophytes will follow. Additional damage that is due to recurrent instability or forced ankle movement, especially forced dorsiflexion, enhances this process. The presence of osteophytes is not always associated with complaints. Asymptomatic ankle osteophytes have been reported in more than 50% of athletes. Arthroscopic removal of symptomatic osteophytes produces good or excellent results in more than 90% of cases [23,24]. Grading of the degenerative changes of the ankle joint in patients who have chronic ankle instability is important for the judgement of the prognosis of ankle joint function in the longer term [24].

Diagnosis of acute ligament injuries

After a supination trauma it is important to distinguish a simple distortion from an acute ankle ligament rupture because adequate treatment is associated with a better prognosis [11]. Because of the often reported poor reliability of physical examination for diagnosis of ligament ruptures after inversion trauma of the ankle, stress radiography, arthrography, MRI, and ultrasonography (US) often are performed simultaneously [23,25]; however, these methods are expensive and their reliability also is debated. The reliability of physical examination can be enhanced when the investigation is repeated a few days after the trauma. The accuracy of physical examination was determined in a series of 160 patients, all of whom underwent arthrography. Physical examination within 48 hours of the injury and 5 days after the injury were compared. The specificity and sensitivity of delayed physical examination for the presence or absence of a lateral ankle ligament rupture were 84% and 96%, respectively. The most important features of physical examination are swelling, hematoma discoloration, pain on palpation, and the anterior drawer test. Physical examination is unreliable in the acute situation; the anterior drawer test cannot be performed because of pain. A few days after the trauma, the swelling and pain have subsided and it becomes obvious if the cause of swelling was edema or hematoma. The pain on palpation has become more localized and the anterior drawer test can now be performed. If there is no pain on palpation over the anterior talo-fibular ligament, there is no acute lateral ligament rupture. Pain on palpation over the anterior talo-fibular ligament itself cannot distinguish between a rupture or a distortion. Pain on palpation, in combination with a hematoma discoloration, has a 90% chance of being an acute lateral ligament rupture. A positive anterior drawer test has a sensitivity of 73% and a specificity of 97%. A positive anterior drawer test, in combination with pain on palpation over the anterior talo-fibular ligament and hematoma discoloration, has a sensitivity of 100% and a specificity of 77%. Delayed physical examination provides a diagnostic modality with a high sensitivity and specificity [5,17,18,26]. It was reported recently by the International Society of Arthroscopy, Knee Surgery and Orthopaedic Sports Medicine consensus meeting to be the method of choice [12].

Treatment of acute ligament injuries

Repeated studies and recent systematic reviews showed that simple sprains can be treated safely nonsurgically. Functional treatment with a short period of rest, cooling (ice), compression, and elevation to reduce the edema (the RICE principle) during the first 1 to 3 days—depending upon the amount of swelling, bruising, and pain—always should be recommended. Early weight bearing without crutches, if possible, is encouraged. Active range of motion training should be started after the acute-phase treatment is completed, followed by neuromuscular coordination training using balance boards and peroneal strengthening exercises [8,27,28].

The injured ligaments should be protected from new injuries during the healing phase by using external support to control the range of motion and to reduce the symptoms of functional instability. Ankle tape and ankle braces (eg, the air-stirrup) are easy to apply, versatile, and effective in stimulating the proprioceptive system. The results of functional treatment of ankle sprains are satisfactory in most cases, and most athletes are able to return to sporting activities within a few weeks [27]. Costs are significantly lower and ankle function is significantly better following early functional brace treatment than after immobilization in a plaster cast [14,29–31].

There is still controversy as to whether ligament ruptures should be treated nonsurgically by active functional treatment and early mobilization, or by primary surgical repair followed by immobilization using a plaster cast or a brace. Only a few prospective, randomized, and controlled studies are found in the literature [32,33]. A recent meta-analysis concluded that surgical treatment leads to superior results in the short- and medium-term follow-up, in terms of giving-way and residual pain. Also, a large, randomized, prospective trial of surgical and functional treatment of lateral ankle ligament ruptures with 6 to 11 years of follow-up revealed that operative treatment leads to less residual pain and giving-way than does functional treatment [34]. Most studies show that the medium- and long-term results are satisfactory in most patients, regardless of the primary choice of treatment (ie, surgical repair, cast immobilization alone for 3–6 weeks, or functional treatment based on the principle of early immobilization). In a prospective, randomized trial that compared early mobilization with plaster cast immobilization, these treatment modalities prevented late residual symptoms and persistent ankle instability equally well; however, patients who were treated with early mobilization had significantly less pain at 3 weeks and were more likely to be back at work after 1 week [29]. Taken together, at least 80% to 90% of patients who have lateral ankle ligament ruptures regain satisfactory functional stability after nonsurgical treatment.

Still, an unsolved problem is how the approximately 30% to 40% of patients who develop chronic instability—despite adequate primary treatment—and may need surgical reconstruction at a later stage, can be identified. Neither the degree of ligament injury nor the degree of radiographic laxity as measured by stress radiographs is a reliable predictor [35].

Ankle joint instability

Functional instability is the most common residual disability after acute, lateral ligament ruptures and is a description of the subjective symptoms of the patient (eg, repeated giving-way, in some cases combined with pain). Conversely, laxity or mechanical instability refers to an objective measurement (eg, standardized stress radiographs, clinical measurement of anterior drawer sign) [36].

Functional instability is a complex syndrome, in which mechanical, neurologic, muscular, and constitutional factors interact. The etiologic factors are not known exactly, and in several cases there is a combination of factors. Elongation of the ruptured ligaments (ie, increased laxity, proprioceptive deficit, peroneal muscle weakness, subtalar instability) is a documented etiologic factor of functional instability, either alone or in combination. Some studies showed a correlation between functional instability and increased laxity using standardized stress radiographs [35,36]. Although these radiographic stress tests may be useful, the reliability of these test is low, and there is no definite correlation between functional instability and increased laxity [9,14,27,28,37].

The reaction time of the peroneal muscles, measured during sudden inversion using an electromyogram, was significantly longer in unstable ankles than in stable ones [37,38]. This difference in the reaction time is due to the time that elapses between the start of the inversion of the ankle and the stimulation of the mechanoreceptors in the ligaments and the joint capsule. Delayed proprioceptive response to a sudden angular displacement of the ankle may be one of the most important causes of functional instability of the ankle joint.

It can be concluded that functional instability is caused by increased laxity, inhibition of proprioceptive function, peroneal muscle weakness, or a combination of these factors. The cause of functional instability has to be analyzed individually.

Chronic ankle instability

Chronic ankle instability develops in approximately 20% of patients after acute ligament rupture [5,6,15]. Ligament laxity does not always require surgical reconstruction. The indication for surgical intervention is recurrent giving-way despite proprioceptive training in patients who have mechanical laxity [8,15,39].

Diagnosis of chronic ankle instability

Clinical tests for acute and chronic ankle instability include the talar tilt test and the anterior drawer test. The talar tilt test is clinically impractical and most often is unreliable [5,10,11] The anterior talo-fibular ligament is the most important stabilizer of the ankle joint. It is the first ligament to rupture during an inversion trauma. Therefore, the anterior drawer test is the most important test for detection of acute and chronic ankle instability [5,11]. Increased anterior translation of the talus in the talo-crural joint can occur when the anterior talo-fibular ligament is ruptured or elongated. There are several ways to perform an anterior drawer test [5]. In most test situations the foot is moved only anteriorly relative to the tibia, and thereby, the ankle is placed in 10° to 20° of plantar flexion. This is an incorrect way to perform the anterior drawer test, and is associated with a higher risk for false-negative test results. The anterior drawer test is not a straightforward translation of the talus in relation to the tibia, but rather it is a rotatory movement [5]. This rotation is caused by the intact deltoid ligament, which prevents the talus from moving forward on the medial side. Therefore, the anterior drawer test should be a combination of a straightforward translation and internal rotation movement (Fig. 2) [28].

Knowledge of the laxity of the ankle joint ligaments in the sagittal and the frontal planes can give valuable information during the diagnostic assessment of chronic functional instability. Radiographic measurements of ankle joint stability are used often before deciding upon the operative treatment of chronic ankle instability [35]. Contrast arthrography and tenography of the peroneal tendons can give concise information on the extent of ligament and tendon injury after acute ruptures; however, these diagnostic tools are hardly necessary and are used rarely [13]. Standardized stress radiographs can be used in the differential diagnostic evaluation and assessment of therapy. Their main drawback is the limited correlation between functional stability and increased laxity.

The lateral instability/laxity test (talar tilt) and the anterior instability/laxity test (anterior talar translation) are the two radiographic tests that are used. Increased laxity can be defined as anterior talar translation of more than 10 mm or

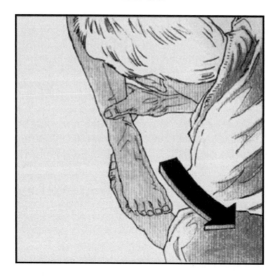

Fig. 2. Anterior drawer test: the foot is pulled anteriorly and medially, using the deltoid ligament as a center of rotation.

talar tilt of more than 9°. Another way of defining increased laxity is a difference in anterior talar translation between the functionally unstable ankle and the contralateral ankle of more than 3 mm, or a talar tilt of more than 3° in patients who have unilateral instability [35,36]. A good correlation between functional and mechanical instability was shown in some studies, but this correlation is highly variable because several factors other than mechanical instability can be responsible for the development of functional instability. Several studies questioned the reliability of stress radiographs, especially the measurements of talar tilt [35,36]. US, CT, and MRI have been used to delineate the extent of damage to the ankle ligaments. US can be useful as a screening modality, especially when there is a discrepancy between clinical and radiologic examinations after trauma. US is inexpensive and noninvasive [23,24]; however, like CT and MRI, it is unable to demonstrate ligament laxity. Both of these modalities, (US, CT and MRI), probably are used little in patients who have chronic ankle instability.

Treatment of chronic ankle instability

Less than 10% of all subjects who sustain acute ligament injuries need stabilizing surgery at a later stage [39]. Before deciding upon surgical treatment in a patient who has chronic ligament insufficiency, a supervised rehabilitation program that is based on peroneal muscle strengthening and coordination training should be completed. More than 50% of patients regain satisfactory functional stability after a 12-week program [29–32]. Patients who have high-grade mechanical laxity have less favorable prospects for regaining satisfactory function after physiotherapy. Surgical treatment should be considered at an earlier stage in these patients.

More than 60 different surgical procedures to stabilize the unstable ankle have been described in the literature. These procedures can be divided into two main groups: tenodesis and anatomic reconstruction.

Tenodesis

Tenodeses were the most widely procedures used in the past. The three classic tenodeses—Evans, Watson-Jones, and Chrisman-Snook—are well documented, and the short- and long-term results are well reported. Of these tenodeses, the Evans tenodesis is the least technically demanding; however, it neither reconstructs the anterior talo-fibular ligament nor the calcaneo-fibular ligament biomechanically, because the tenodesis is positioned in a plane between these two ligaments. Several investigators reported good short-term results after this reconstruction and its modifications, but the long-term results have varied. Many patients' early satisfactory results deteriorated after a few years, which resulted in unsatisfactory function in the long run. In one study, less than 50% of subjects had satisfactory results after a mean follow-up period of 14 years [40]. The Watson-Jones tenodesis reconstructs the anterior talofibular ligament, but not the calcaneo-fibular ligament. Several good short-term results have been reported, but long-term follow-up studies showed disappointing functional results in approximately two thirds of the patients [40–43]. Late deterioration is common, with increased laxity and reduction of ankle function, as well as pain. The Chrisman-Snook tenodesis restores the anterior talo-fibular ligament and the calcaneo-fibular ligament, and probably is the most widely used nonanatomic reconstruction (Fig. 3)

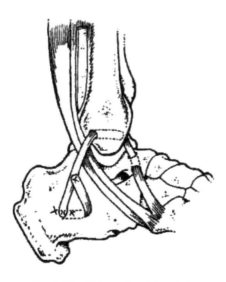

Fig. 3. The Chrisman-Snook tenodesis.

[44]. The peroneus brevis tendon is split longitudinally, and half of the tendon is used to reconstruct both ligaments. In one study, satisfactory results were reported in 94% of patients [43]. Stress provocation also showed less residual laxity after the Chrisman-Snook reconstruction than after the Evans reconstruction. The Chrisman-Snook procedure is more demanding technically than are the other tenodeses.

One of the major drawbacks is that all tenodeses are nonanatomic reconstructions and they sacrifice normal, and in most cases, well-functioning anatomic structures around the ankle joint (ie, the peroneus brevis or peroneus longus tendons). This results in altered kinematics, often limitation of joint motion and gradual deterioration of the reconstructed ligament function [45]. The consequence could be the development of degenerative changes of the ankle in the long run [46,47]. All of these procedures can restrict the subtalar motion. Biomechanical analysis of nonanatomic reconstructions showed that ligamentous isometricity is lacking and that normal ankle biomechanics are not restored [48].

Complications after a nonanatomic reconstruction procedure have been reported. Most complications are related to the long skin incision that is needed for harvesting the peroneus brevis tendon. Problems with delayed wound healing and sural nerve injuries also have been described [49,50].

Unlike anatomic reconstruction, tenodesis does not restore the normal anatomy of the lateral ankle ligaments. These procedures result in a restricted range of ankle motion, a higher number of reoperations, impairment of athletic performance, and unsatisfactory functional results [45,46,51]. Furthermore, many studies reported that tenodesis does not prevent mechanical laxity entirely, and thereby, leads to subsequent degenerative changes on the medial side of the ankle joint [47].

Because of the elongation or loosening of the tendon in the long term, the restriction in the range of ankle motion resolves and mechanical instability becomes more persistent. This leads to the development of more severe degenerative changes in the ankle joint. Subsequently, the risk for the development of osteophytes and the need for a reoperative procedure to remove these osteophytes increases over time. Therefore, anatomic reconstruction of the lateral ankle ligaments can be regarded as the surgical treatment of choice in patients who have chronic ankle instability [45–47,51]; however, tenodesis can play a role in secondary procedures.

Anatomic reconstruction

The basic principle of anatomic reconstruction is to restore the normal anatomic ligamentous proportions, which should lead to the original biomechanical situation of the lateral ligament complex of the ankle joint. Anatomic reconstruction of the anterior talo-fibular ligament is simple. The insertion at the tip of the fibula and the talus is uniform. Most anatomy textbooks describe the existence of a single anterior talo-fibular ligament. In a certain percentage (~10–30%) of patients, anatomically as well as functionally, upper and lower parts of the ligament may be distinguished [5]. The insertion of the calcaneo-fibular ligament at the tip of the fibula also is uniform. It arises from the anterior part and runs obliquely downward and backward to attach to the lateral surface of the calcaneus. This insertion point is less unambiguous. In the plantigrade foot there is interindividual direction of the calcaneo-fibular ligament, which lies between 10° and 80° posteriorly. There also is a considerable interindividual variety in the length of the calcaneo-fibular ligament [2,5]. After a rupture of this ligament it is difficult to identify its original insertion at the calcaneus. Therefore, it is doubtful whether anatomic reconstruction of the calcaneo-fibular ligament is possible. An anatomic reconstruction is a reconstruction in which a ligament is restored to its original insertions.

Anatomic reconstructions can be classified into four categories:

Anatomic reconstruction using the original ligament remnants
Anatomic reconstruction using the original ligament ends with reinforcement
    of local tissues (eg, periosteum, inferior extensor retinaculum)
Anatomic reconstruction using an autograft
Anatomic reconstruction using an allograft

Anatomic reconstruction using the original ligament remnants

Broström [2], who described this procedure in detail, found that direct suture (repair) of the ruptured and elongated ligaments was possible, even several years after the primary injury. The combination of shortening, imbrication, and reinsertion to the bony attachment of the injured ligaments has been successful [52]. Satisfactory functional results after anatomic reconstruction of the lateral ankle ligaments were described in several studies [8,39,51–54]. The surgical technique is simple and is performed easily. The damaged or elongated remnants of the anterior talo-fibular ligament and calcaneo-fibular ligament are divided, shortened 3 mm to 5 mm, imbricated, and reinserted into bone (Fig. 4).

Satisfactory functional results were reported in approximately 90% of patients, with radiographic evidence of less residual laxity [39,49,52]. The results are less satisfactory in patients who have generalized hypermobility of the joints or long-standing ligamentous insufficiency (>10 years), and in patients who have undergone previous ankle joint ligament surgery.

Anatomic reconstruction using the original ligament ends is technically simple, gives rise to few complications, and produces short- and long-term satisfactory functional results [45–47,51].

Anatomic reconstruction using the original ligament ends with reinforcement of local tissues

In some cases, the original ligament ends are too weak or too damaged to perform a sufficient reconstruction; local structures can be used for reinforcement. These modifications include using a periosteal flap from the lateral aspect of the fibula and the inferior extensor retinaculum, and reinforcement of the calcaneo-fibular ligament repair with the lateral talo-calcaneal ligament [54,55].

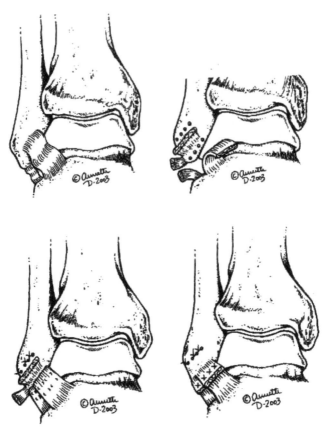

Fig. 4. Shortening, imbrication, and reinsertion of the anterior talo-fibular ligament and calcaneo-fibular ligament.

Also, tensioning of the lateral ankle ligaments and capsular tissue has been described. Experimental studies reported that the use of these structures do not disturb normal joint kinematics [50,56,57].

Anatomic reconstruction using an autograft

Another principle of anatomic reconstruction is reconstruction using an autograft. In 1968, Weber described a procedure in which the anterior talo-fibular ligament is reconstructed using the plantaris tendon [58]. The plantaris tendon can be detached with a stripper. Holes are drilled on the original insertions of the anterior talo-fibular ligament at the fibula and the talus. The graft is pulled through these holes in a figure-eight loop. It mimics, to some extent, the situation in patients who have an anterior talo-fibular ligament that is built out of two separate bundles. Segesser and Goesele [58] described a modification of the Weber procedure by which the anterior talo-fibular ligament and calcaneo-fibular ligament are reconstructed.

Other examples of autografts for anatomic reconstruction are the Achilles tendon, as in the Solheim procedure, and the use of free fascia lata that was described by Elmslie in 1934 [58]. These procedures are used rarely today.

Anatomic reconstruction using an allograft

The use of fresh frozen allografts in the reconstruction of the lateral ankle ligaments gave satisfactory results in one study. Neither immunologic rejections nor complaints of late instability was reported [56]. Because no normal tissues are sacrificed, this procedure can be considered as an alternative if the quality of the ligamentous tissue is poor.

Arthroscopic ligament stabilization

Arthroscopic ligament stabilization was reported to be an alternative to open reconstructions [59]. The anterior talo-fibular ligament is shortened and reinserted by the use of a percutaneous staple. Only a few reports on this technique are found in the literature and it probably is used rarely today. There might be a specific indication for this technique in children to avoid damage to the growth plate of the fibula. A drawback of the arthroscopic stabilization is that this technique makes it possible to reconstruct only the anterior talo-fibular ligament.

Arthroscopic thermal capsular shrinkage is a recently developed alternative method for the treatment of chronic joint instability. Originally, shrinkage was performed with a laser, but the radiofrequency thermal probe seems to be more appropriate because of the better-controlled method of application. Different investigators reported their results, mainly in experimental cadaver and biomechanical studies and in clinical studies with patients who suffered from shoulder instability. Cadaver studies showed that shrinkage of ligaments of up to 30% can be reached. Biomechanical studies showed that there is an initial susceptibility to creep after shrinkage; however, remodelling is complete and normal tissue strength is regained after 6 to 12 weeks [60].

The treatment of chronic knee and shoulder instability with thermal capsular shrinkage shows a high failure rate [61]. Only a combination of sutures and shrinkage seems to lead to acceptable results [62].

The biomechanics of the ankle are different from those of the shoulder and the knee. Intrinsically, the ankle is the most stable joint of the body, which makes its functional stability less dependent on the ligaments and joint capsule. Therefore, the chronically unstable ankle is a better candidate for treatment with arthroscopic capsular shrinkage. Furthermore, the anterolateral ankle ligaments, as capsular structures, are easily accessible by the electrocoagulation device under arthroscopic vision. The mean length of the elongated anterior talo-fibular ligament is 30 mm, whereas its mean normal length is 20 mm (Fig. 5). With 30% shrinkage, the original length of the ligament can be regained.

Oloff and colleagues [63] performed a study that treated 10 patients who had chronic lateral ankle instability using arthroscopic monopolar radiofrequency thermal shrinkage. Their results were encouraging; patients returned to full ac-

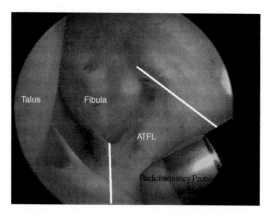

Fig. 5. Arthroscopic view of the anterolateral gutter of a left ankle: shrinkage of the anterior talofibular ligament (ATFL) is performed with the radiofrequency probe.

tivity in 3 months and all patients achieved ankle stability. Berlet and colleagues [64] performed a comparable study with 16 patients, with good to excellent result in 80% of the patients. The authors are conducting a multicenter study that includes almost 40 patients who have chronic ankle instability. The preliminary results show that arthroscopic thermal capsular shrinkage is a safe method, and that functional stability is improved in most patients. Improvement of mechanical stability is less evident. Future studies should answer the question of whether there is a permanent mechanical improvement—and if that is not the case—what is the alternative explanation for the functional improvement.

Subtalar instability

Subtalar instability lacks a well-established clinical and scientific definition. Despite this, ligament insufficiency of the subtalar joints can be regarded as one of the factors behind the development of chronic functional instability. The ligaments of the subtalar joint consist of three layers within the sinus and canalis tarsi and the lateral aspect of the subtalar joint [65]. The prevalence of subtalar instability is unknown. Most injuries occur in combination with injuries of the lateral ankle ligaments. Subtalar instability has an estimated prevalence of 10% in patients who have chronic lateral ankle instability, but is not well proven scientifically [65,66]. Using subtalar arthrography, injuries to the subtalar joints have been found in a high proportion of patients who have sustained acute lateral ligament injuries [66]. The clinical diagnosis of subtalar instability is difficult and unreliable. The diagnosis can be supported by using subtalar arthrography, subtalar stress radiographs, or stress tomography. The value of MRI, CT, and US in the diagnostic evaluation of subtalar instability is unknown, and only a few studies in the literature concern the diagnostic assessment and therapeutic methods. Analysis of the degree of disability that is related to subtalar instability is lacking.

Anatomic reconstruction is recommended in patients who have chronic instability of subtalar joints that does not respond to a supervised rehabilitation program. The superficial layer of the inferior extensor retinaculum can be used to bridge the subtalar joint. The short-term results of these procedures are promising, but further studies are needed to evaluate the long-lasting function objectively [66]. Another option is a tenodesis procedure that bridges the subtalar joint. These procedures, however, are nonanatomic and lead to limitation of the subtalar joint motion. No comparative studies are found, which implies that the optimal treatment is still unknown.

Summary

Unlike anatomic reconstruction, tenodesis does not restore the normal anatomy of the lateral ankle ligaments. These procedures result in a restricted range of ankle motion, a higher number of reoperations, impairment of athletic performance, and unsatisfactory functional results. Tenodesis does not prevent mechanical laxity entirely, and thereby, leads to subsequent degenerative changes on the medial side of the ankle joint.

Because of the elongation or loosening of the tendon in the long-term, the restriction in the range of ankle motion resolves and mechanical instability becomes more persistent. This leads to the development of more severe degenerative changes in the ankle joint. Subsequently, the risk for the development of osteophytes and the need for a reoperative procedure to remove these osteophytes increases over time.

Anatomic reconstruction of the lateral ankle ligaments can be regarded as the surgical treatment of choice in patients who have ankle instability. Even when the original ligament ends are absent or too weak to perform a sufficient reconstruction, alternative procedures, such as reinforcement with local tissues or the augmentation of autografts, have been developed to overcome this problem.

There are some remaining issues concerning anatomic reconstruction. Because the insertion of the calcaneo-fibular ligament at the calcaneus shows a high interindividual variety, it is doubtful whether reconstruction of this ligament is truly anatomic. Several studies reported that reconstruction of the anterior talo-fibular ligament and the calcaneo-fibular ligament improve the results. When we are able to identify the original calcaneal insertion of the calcaneo-fibular ligament, theoretically we will be able to restore the original direction of this ligament, and thus, not disturb isometricity. More experimental and clinical studies are needed to solve this issue.

The role of the subtalar joint in the etiology of ankle instability remains unclear. Pathologic instability of the subtalar joint is not defined clearly, and probably is difficult to objectify. Most studies that deal with ankle instability aim at outcome measures that concern the function and state of the ankle joint. A reconstructive procedure, especially when it includes reconstruction of the calcaneo-fibular ligament, inevitably influences the subtalar joint as well. This remains ignored to some degree in the literature and needs clarification.

Another problem is that the development of degenerative changes is not prevented by anatomic reconstruction. Therefore, a short interval (ie, <6 months) between the onset of symptomatic instability and the reconstructive procedure is recommended.

As with any open surgical procedure, anatomic reconstruction is correlated with the risk for infection, hematoma, nerve damage, and postoperative dystrophy. The role of minimally invasive procedures, such as arthroscopic stapling repair and thermal capsular shrinkage, in the treatment of chronic ankle instability have yet to be established.

Acknowledgments

We thank Annette Dahlstrom for the preparation of Figs. 1 through 4.

References

[1] Wiersman PH, Grifioen FMM. Variations of three lateral ligaments of the ankle. A descriptive anatomical study. Foot 1992;2:218–22.

[2] Broström L. Sprained ankles: a pathologic, arthrographic and clinical study [doctoral dissertation]. Stockholm: Karolinska Institute; 1966.

[3] Rasmussen O, Kromann-Andersen C. Experimental ankle injuries. Analysis of the traumatology of the ankle ligaments. Acta Orthop Scand 1983;54:356–62.

[4] Fallat L, Grimm DJ, Saracco JA. Sprained ankle syndrome: prevalence and analysis of 639 acute injuries. J Foot Ankle Surg 1998;37:280–5.

[5] Van Dijk CN. On diagnostic strategies in patients with severe ankle sprain [master's thesis]. Amsterdam: Universiteit van Amsterdam; 1994.

[6] Kannus P, Renström P. Treatment for acute tears of the lateral ligaments of the ankle. Operation, cast, or early controlled mobilization. J Bone Joint Surg Am 1991;73:305–12.

[7] Klenerman L. The management of sprained ankle. J Bone Joint Surg Br 1998;80:11–2.

[8] Hamilton WG. Current concepts in the treatment of acute and chronic lateral ligament instability. Sports Medicine and Arthroscopic Review 1994;2:264–71.

[9] Konradsen L, Hölmer P, Söndergaard L. Early mobilizing treatment for grade III ankle ligament injuries. Foot Ankle 1991;12:69–73.

[10] Van Dijk CN. CBO-guideline for diagnosis and treatment of the acute ankle injury. National organization for quality assurance in hospitals. Ned Tijdschr Geneeskd 1999;143:2097–101.

[11] Van Dijk CN, Lim LS, Bossuyt PM, et al. Physical examination is sufficient for the diagnosis of sprained ankles. J Bone Joint Surg Br 1996;78:958–62.

[12] International Society of Arthroscopy, Knee Surgery and Orthopaedic Sports Medicine— International Federation of Sports Medicine (ISAKOS–FIMS). World Consensus Conference on Ankle Instability. Editors: KM Chan & Jon Karlsson. C. Niek van Dijk. Diagnosis of ankle sprain: history and physical examination. 21–22, January 2005.

[13] Prins JG. Diagnosis and treatment of injury to the lateral ligament of the ankle. A comparative clinical study. Acta Chir Scand Suppl 1978;486:3–149.

[14] Karlsson J, Andreasson GO. The effect of external ankle support in chronic lateral ankle joint instability An electromyographic study. Am J Sports Med 1992;20:257–61.

[15] Karlsson J, Lansinger O. Lateral instability of the ankle joint. Clin Orthop Rel Res 1992;276: 253 – 61.

[16] Fritschy D. An unusual ankle injury in top skiers. Am J Sports Med 1989;17:282 – 5.

[17] Boytim MJ, Fischer DA, Neumann L. Syndesmotic ankle sprains. Am J Sports Med 1991;19: 294 – 8.

[18] Taylor DC, Englehardt DL, Bassett III FH. Syndesmosis sprains of the ankle. The influence of heterotopic ossification. Am J Sports Med 1992;20:146 – 50.

[19] Hopkinson WJ, St Pierre P, Ryan JB, et al. Syndesmosis sprains of the ankle. Foot Ankle 1990;10:325 – 30.

[20] Xenos JS, Hopkinson WJ, Mulligan ME, et al. The tibiofibular syndesmosis. Evaluation of the ligamentous structures, methods of fixation, and radiographic assessment. J Bone Joint Surg Am 1995;77:847 – 56.

[21] Kiter E, Bozkurt M. The crossed-leg test for examination of ankle syndesmosis injuries. Foot Ankle Int 2005;26(2):187 – 8.

[22] Van Dijk CN, Bossuyt PM, Marti RK. Medial ankle pain after lateral ligament rupture. J Bone Joint Surg Br 1996;78:562 – 7.

[23] Tol JL, Verheyen CP, van Dijk CN. Arthroscopic treatment of anterior impingement in the ankle. J Bone Joint Surg Br 2001;83:9 – 13.

[24] Van Dijk CN, Tol JL, Verheyen CC. A prospective study of prognostic factors concerning the outcome of arthroscopic surgery for anterior ankle impingement. Am J Sports Med 1997;25: 737 – 45.

[25] Friedrich JM, Schnarkowski P, Rübenacker S, et al. Ultrasonography of capsular morphology in normal and traumatic ankle joints. J Clin Ultrasound 1993;21:179 – 87.

[26] Van Dijk CN, Mol BW, Lim LS, et al. Diagnosis of ligament rupture of the ankle joint. Physical examination, arthrography, stress radiography, and sonography compared in 160 patients after inversion trauma. Acta Orthop Scand 1996;67:566 – 70.

[27] Kerkhoffs GM, Struijs PA, Marti RK, et al. Functional treatments for acute ruptures of the lateral ankle ligament: a systematic review. Acta Orthop Scand 2003;74(1):69 – 77.

[28] Kerkhoffs GM, Blankevoort L, Sierevelt IN, et al. Two ankle joint laxity testers: reliability and validity. Knee Surg Sports Traumatol Arthrosc 2005;13(8):699 – 705.

[29] Karlsson J, Lansinger O, Faxén E. Conservative treatment of chronic lateral instability of the ankle. Swedish Medical Journal 1991;88:1404 – 7.

[30] Kerkhoffs GM, Rowe BH, Assendelft WJ, et al. Immobilisation and functional treatment for acute lateral ankle ligament injuries in adults. Cochrane Database Syst Rev 2002;3:CD003762.

[31] Kerkhoffs GM, Rowe BH, Assendelft WJ, et al. Immobilisation for acute ankle sprain. A systematic review. Arch Orthop Trauma Surg 2001;121:462 – 71.

[32] Munk B, Holm-Christensen K, Lind T. Long-term outcome after ruptured lateral ankle ligaments. A prospective study of three different treatments in 79 patients with 11-year follow-up. Acta Orthop Scand 1995;66:452 – 4.

[33] Povacz P, Unger SF, Miller WK, et al. A randomized, prospective study of operative and non-operative treatment of injuries of the fibular collateral ligaments of the ankle. J Bone Joint Surg Am 1998;80:345 – 51.

[34] Pijnenburg ACM, van Dijk CN, Bossuyt PM, et al. Treatment for lateral ankle ligament ruptures: a meta-analysis. J Bone Joint Surg Am 2000;82:761 – 73.

[35] Karlsson J. Chronic lateral instability of the ankle joint: a clinical, radiological and experimental study [doctoral dissertation]. Gothenburg (Sweden): Gothenburg University; 1989.

[36] Karlsson J, Bergsten T, Peterson L, et al. Radiographic evaluation of ankle joint stability. Clinical Journal of Sports Medicine 1991;1:166 – 71.

[37] Karlsson J, Peterson L, Andreasson GO, et al. The unstable ankle: a combined EMG and biomechanical modeling study. Int J Sports Biomechanics 1992;8:129 – 34.

[38] Konradsen L, Ravn JB, Sörensen AI. Proprioception at the ankle: The effect of anesthetic blockade of ligament receptors. J Bone Joint Surg Br 1993;75:433 – 6.

[39] Karlsson J, Bergsten T, Lansinger O, et al. Reconstruction of the lateral ligaments of the ankle for chronic lateral instability. J Bone Joint Surg Am 1988;70:581 – 8.

[40] Karlsson J, Bergsten T, Lansinger O, et al. Lateral instability of the ankle treated by the Evans procedure: a long-term clinical and radiological follow-up. J Bone Joint Surg Br 1988;70: 476–80.

[41] Rosenbaum D, Becker HP, Sterk J, et al. Long-term results of the modified Evans repair for chronic ankle instability. Orthopedics 1996;18:451–5.

[42] Rosenbaum D, Becker HP, Sterk J, et al. Functional evaluation of the 10-year outcome after modified Evans repair for chronic ankle instability. Foot Ankle Int 1997;18:765–71.

[43] Snook GA, Chrisman OD, Wilson TC. Long-term results of the Chrisman-Snook operation for reconstruction of the lateral ligaments of the ankle. J Bone Joint Surg Am 1985;67:1–7.

[44] Hennrikus WL, Mapes RC, Lyons PM, et al. Outcomes of the Chrisman Snook and modified Broström procedures for chronic lateral ankle instability. A prospective, randomized comparison. Am J Sports Med 1996;24:400–4.

[45] Krips R, van Dijk CN, Lehtonen H, et al. Sports activity level after surgical treatment for chronic anterolateral ankle instability: a multicenter study. Am J Sports Med 2002;30(1):13–9.

[46] Krips R, van Dijk CN, Halasi T, et al. Long-term outcome of anatomical reconstruction versus tenodesis for the treatment of chronic anterolateral instability of the ankle joint; a multicenter study. Foot Ankle Int 2001;22(5):415–21.

[47] Krips R, Brandsson S, Svensson C, et al. Anatomical reconstruction and Evans tenodesis of the lateral ligaments of the ankle. Clinical and radiological findings after follow-up for 15 to 30 years. J Bone Joint Surg Br 2002;84(2):232–6.

[48] Rosenbaum D, Becker HP, Wilke HJ, et al. Tenodeses destroy the kinematic coupling of the ankle joint complex: a three-dimensional in vitro analysis of joint movement. J Bone Joint Surg Br 1998;80:162–8.

[49] Mabit C, Chaudruc JM, Fiorenza F, et al. Lateral ligament of the ankle: comparative study of peroneus brevis tenodesis versus periosteal ligamentoplasty. Foot Ankle Surg 1998;4:71–6.

[50] Liu SH, Baker CL. Comparison of lateral ankle ligamentous reconstruction procedures. Am J Sports Med 1993;22:313–7.

[51] Krips R, van Dijk CN, Halasi T, et al. Anatomical reconstruction versus tenodesis for the treatment of chronic anterolateral ankle instability; a 2- to 10- year follow-up, multi-center study. Knee Surg Sports Traumatol Arthrosc 2000;8(3):173–9.

[52] Karlsson J, Bergsten T, Lansinger O, et al. Surgical treatment of chronic lateral instability of the ankle joint: a new procedure. Am J Sports Med 1989;17:268–73.

[53] Sjölin SU, Dons-Jensen H, Simonsen O. Reinforced anatomical reconstruction of the anterior talo-fibular ligament in chronic anterolateral instability using a periosteal flap. Foot Ankle 1991; 12:15–8.

[54] Rudert M, Wülker N, Wirth CJ. Reconstruction of the lateral ligaments of the ankle using a regional periosteal flap. J Bone Joint Surg Br 1997;79:446–51.

[55] Saragaglia D, Fontanel F, Montbaron E, et al. Reconstruction of the lateral ankle ligaments using an inferior extensor retinaculum flap. Foot Ankle Int 1997;18:723–8.

[56] Becker HP, Rosenbaum D, Ziethammel G, et al. Tenodesis versus carbon fiber repair of ankle ligaments. A clinical comparison. Clin Orthop Rel Res 1996;325:194–202.

[57] Bahr R, Pena F, Shine J, et al. Biomechanics of ankle ligament reconstruction. An in vitro comparison of the Broström repair, Watson-Jones reconstruction, and a new anatomic reconstruction technique. Am J Sports Med 1997;25:424–32.

[58] Segesser B, Goesele A. Weber fibular ligament-plasty with plantar tendon with Segesser modification. Sportverletz Sportschaden 1996;10:88–93.

[59] Hawkins RB. Arthroscopic stapling repair for chronic lateral instability. Clin Pod Med Surg 1987;4:875–83.

[60] Lu Y, Hayashi K, Fanton GS, et al. the effect of monopolar radiofrequency treatment pattern on joint capsular healing. In vitro and in vivo studies using an ovine model. Am J Sports Med 2000;28:711–9.

[61] D'Allesandro DF, Bradley JP, Fleischli JE, et al. Prospective evaluation of thermal capsulorrhaphy for shoulder instability. Am J Sport Med 2004;32:21–33.

[62] Bohnsack M, Ruhmann O, Hurschler C, et al. Arthroscopic anterior shoulder stabilization: combined multiple suture repair and laser-assisted capsular shrinkage. Injury 2002;33:795–9.

[63] Oloff LM, Bocko AP, Fanton G. Arthroscopic monopolar radiofrequency thermal stabilization for chronic lateral ankle instability: a preliminary report on 10 cases. J Foot Ankle Surg 2000; 39:144–53.

[64] Berlet GC, Saar WE, Ryan A, et al. Thermal-assisted capsular modification for functional ankle instability. Foot Ankle Clin 2002;7:567–76.

[65] Harper MC. The lateral ligamentous support of the subtalar joint. Foot Ankle 1991;11:354–8.

[66] Schon LC, Clanton TO, Baxter DE. Reconstruction for subtalar instability: a review. Foot Ankle 1991;11:319–24.

ELSEVIER
SAUNDERS

Foot Ankle Clin N Am
11 (2006) 331–359

FOOT AND
ANKLE CLINICS

Current Concepts: Treatment of Osteochondral Ankle Defects

Maartje Zengerink, MD[a],*, Imre Szerb, MD, PhD[b],
László Hangody, MD, PhD, DSc[b], Ryan M. Dopirak, MD[c],
Richard D. Ferkel, MD[c], C. Niek van Dijk, MD, PhD, DSc[a]

[a]Department of Orthopaedic Surgery, Academic Medical Center, University of Amsterdam,
P.O. Box 22660, 1100 DD Amsterdam, The Netherlands
[b]Uzsoki Hospital, Department of Orthopaedics, Mexikói Street 64, 1145 Budapest, Hungary
[c]Southern California Orthopedic Institute, 6815 Noble Avenue, Van Nuys, CA 91405, USA

An osteochondral lesion of the talus (OLT) is a lesion involving talar articular cartilage and subchondral bone mostly caused by a traumatic event, leading to partial or complete detachment of the osteochondral fragment, with or without osteonecrosis.

Many terms are in use, including osteochondral fracture, osteochondral lesion, osteochondritis dissecans, transchondral fracture, flake fracture, and intra-articular fracture.

Osteochondral defects can occur in any joint. The most common location is the knee. Osteochondral defects of the ankle account for approximately 4% of the total number of osteochondral defects [1]. Osteochondral defects of the ankle occur most frequently in 20- to 30-year-old men [2]. Defects can be found on the medial and lateral sides of the talar dome, and occasionally are located centrally [3].

In 1856, Monro first reported the presence of cartilaginous bodies in the (ankle) joint [3a]. In 1870, Paget further described the defects [4], and in 1888, König [4a] first used the term osteochondritis dissecans for loose body formation associated with articular cartilage and subchondral bone fracture in the knee. König [4a] suggested that these loose bodies were the result of spontaneous osteonecrosis secondary to vascular occlusion of the subchondral bone. He used

---

* Corresponding author.
E-mail address: m.zengerink@amc.uva.nl (M. Zengerink).

the term *osteochondritis* to refer to an inflammatory process, and *dissecans*, derived from the Latin word *dissecare*, to separate. Involvement of an inflammatory process in the pathology, however, has never been proved.

Rendu [5], in 1932, also described the condition. Davidson and colleagues [6], Flick and Gould [7], and Nash and Baker [8] discussed the late finding of OLT after an initially diagnosed "sprained ankle." Canale and Belding [9] further emphasized trauma as a causative factor.

Concerning trauma, it is estimated that one ankle injury per 10,000 people per day occurs [10]. Ankle injuries compose 45% of basketball injuries, 25% of volleyball injuries, and 31% of football injuries [11]. The percentage of osteochondral lesions associated with lateral ankle ligament rupture was determined by three investigators who routinely inspected the lateral talar dome in a consecutive series of patients who were operated for lateral ankle ligament rupture. Bosien and colleagues [12], van Dijk [13], and Lippert and colleagues [14] respectively reported 5%, 6%, and 9% lateral talar dome lesions. The percentage of medial dome lesions is unknown but estimated to be as high as lateral talar dome lesions [13].

Lateral lesions cause more symptoms than medial ones. When the lesion is large and the affected piece is dissected, the joint mechanics are altered, which may lead to osteoarthritis.

In 1959, Berndt and Harty [15] gave the first classification determined by radiographic appearance (Box 1); however, the diagnostic approach is based on MRI or CT findings, and different classifications have been made [16–19].

An osteochondral lesion of the trochlea tali is often not recognized as such and, therefore, not adequately treated. Nonrecognition is mainly due to the fact that the lesion can remain asymptomatic or produce symptoms of inversion–distorsion. To a lesser degree, nonrecognition is also due to the fact that an osteochondral defect often cannot be identified on a plain radiograph. After standard treatment for acute ankle sprains, residual symptoms are reported in 33% to 40% of patients [12]. When symptoms persist after an ankle sprain, the possibility of an osteochondral defect needs to be considered.

Box 1. Grading system for osteochondral ankle lesions

Stage I: a small compression fracture
Stage II: incomplete avulsion of a fragment
Stage III: complete avulsion of a fragment without displacement
Stage IV: displaced fragment

(*Adapted from* Berndt AL, Harty M. Transchondral fractures (osteochondritis dissecans) of the talus. J Bone Joint Surg Am 1959;41: 1005; with permission. Copyright is owned by the *Journal of Bone and Joint Surgery*.)

Therapeutic results can be improved by earlier diagnosis and more adequate treatment of the condition. During the past 10 years, great development has been seen in the field of OLT treatment.

The aim of this article is to provide an overview of osteochondral ankle defects, including symptoms and specific treatment indications. Three operative techniques are highlighted: debridement and bone marrow stimulation, osteochondral transplants, and autologous chondrocyte implantation.

Etiology

Traumatic insult is more widely accepted as the etiology of OLTs, although not without controversy. It is likely that trauma and ischemia are both involved in the pathology. Because not all patients report a history of ankle injury, a subdivision can be made in the etiology of nontraumatic and traumatic defects.

The nontraumatic etiology concerns idiopathic osteochondral defects. In these defects, ischemia, subsequent necrosis, and possibly genetics are etiologic factors. Osteochondral defects in identical twins and in siblings have been described [20–22]. In 10% to 25% of patients, the occurrence of the defect is bilateral [9,15].

In the etiology of traumatic osteochondral defects, ankle sprains play the largest role. A severe ankle sprain can cause a small fracture and subsequent impaired vascularity, leading to the formation of an osteochondral defect. In addition, microtraumas caused by repetitive articular cartilage surface loading or excessive stress can lead to cellular degeneration or death by the disruption of collagen fibril ultrastructure and thickening of the subchondral bone [23].

In lateral lesions, trauma is described in 98% of cases; in medial lesions, trauma is described in 70% [7].

Mechanism of injury

When the talus twists inside its boxlike housing during an ankle sprain, the cartilage lining can be damaged. It may lead to a bruise and subsequent softening of the cartilage or worse: a crack in the cartilage or delamination. Separation of the cartilage can occur in the upper layer as a result of shearing forces. Alternatively, separation may occur in the subchondral bone, giving rise to a subchondral lesion. Fragments can break off and float loose in the ankle joint or they can remain partially attached and in position. Progression may result in increased joint pressure, resulting in the forcing of synovial fluid into the epiphysis, creating a subchondral cyst. The subchondral cyst and increased joint pressure may prevent healing. The subchondral fracture has no soft tissue attachments and is highly susceptible to subsequent avascular necrosis.

In cadaver ankles, Berndt and Harty [15] reproduced lateral defects by strongly inverting a dorsiflexed ankle. As the foot was inverted on the leg, the

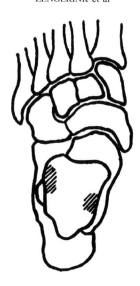

Fig. 1. Main locations of osteochondral ankle defects: the anterolateral and posteromedial talar dome.

lateral border of the talar dome was compressed against the face of the fibula. When the lateral ligament ruptured, avulsion of the chip began. This chip could be completely detached and remain in place or be displaced by supination. With the use of excessive inverting force, the talus within the mortise was rotated laterally in the frontal plane, impacting and compressing the lateral talar margin against the articular surface of the fibula. A portion of the talar margin was sheared off from the main body of the talus, which caused a lateral osteochondral defect. These investigators were able to reproduce a medial lesion by plantar flexing the ankle, by performing a slight anterior displacement of the talus on the tibia, by inversion, and by internal rotation of the talus on the tibia.

Lateral osteochondral lesions are usually located in the anterior third of the talar dome, and medial lesions are mostly located in the posterior half (Fig. 1); however, there are exceptions, and anteromedial, posterolateral, and centrally located lesions may occur after trauma. An individual may have multiple lesions. The lateral lesions are typically shallow and wafer-shaped, indicating a shear mechanism of injury. In contrast, medial lesions are generally deep and cup-shaped, indicating a mechanism of torsional impaction. Medial lesions are usually asymmetric, whereas lateral lesions are symmetric. Because of their shape, lateral lesions are more often displaced than medial lesions.

Clinical presentation

A differentiation has to be made between the acute and the chronic situation. In the acute situation, symptoms of osteochondral ankle defects compare with those of acute ankle injuries. They include lateral or medial ankle pain, swelling, and limited range of motion. In patients who have an isolated ligamentous ankle injury, these symptoms usually resolve after functional treatment within 2 to 3 weeks. If symptoms do not resolve after 3 to 6 weeks, an (osteo)chondral defect of the talus should be suspected. These patients typically present with persisting symptoms and a limited range of motion.

Locking and catching are symptoms of a displaced fragment. In most patients who have a nondisplaced lesion after supination trauma, the symptoms in the acute situation cannot be distinguished from the soft tissue damage.

Chronic lesions classically present as deep lateral or medial ankle pain associated with weight bearing. Reactive swelling and stiffness can be present, but absence of swelling, locking, or catching does not rule out an osteochondral defect. Recognizable pain on palpation is typically not present in these patients. Some patients have diminished range of motion.

Diagnosis

After careful history taking and physical examination of the ankle, routine radiographs of the ankle are taken, consisting of weight bearing anteroposterior, mortise, and lateral views of both ankles.

The radiographs may show an area of detached bone surrounded by radio-lucency (Fig. 2). Initially, the damage may be too small to be visualized on routine radiography. By repeating the imaging studies in a later stage, the abnormality sometimes becomes apparent.

A heelrise view with the ankle in a plantar-flexed position may reveal a posteromedial or posterolateral defect [24]. A bone scan can differentiate between a symptomatic lesion and an asymptomatic lesion. MRI is often used for detection of these lesions. CT is useful for better defining the exact size and location of the lesion and, therefore, more valuable for preoperative planning

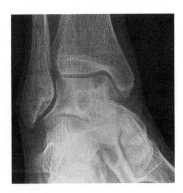

Fig. 2. Plain anteroposterior radiograph of the ankle: radiolucency of the medial talar dome indicating an osteochondral defect.

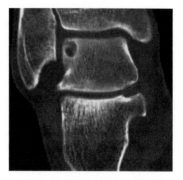

Fig. 3. CT scan of a lateral osteochondral ankle defect; coronal reconstruction.

(Figs. 3 and 4). In diagnosing an osteochondral defect, CT has proved to be equally as valuable as MRI [24].

Operative treatment options

There are widely published surgical techniques for treatment of symptomatic osteochondral lesions. Generally, these techniques are based on one of the following three principles [25–32]:

1. Debridement and bone marrow stimulation, potentially in combination with loose body removal (microfracture, abrasion arthroplasty, or drilling)
2. Securing a lesion to the talar dome (retrograde drilling, bone grafting, or internal fixation)
3. Stimulating the development of hyaline cartilage (osteochondral autografts [mosaicplasty], allografts, or autologous chondrocyte implantation [ACI])

Assessment of the lesion and possible surgical approaches are significant issues when dealing with OLTs. In Parisien's [30] comprehensive report on ankle arthroscopy techniques, he described portal approaches for synovectomy, debridement, loose body removal, curettage, abrasion, and drilling in the treat-

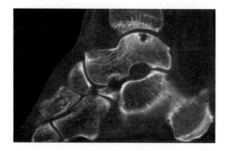

Fig. 4. CT scan of a medial osteochondral ankle defect; sagittal reconstruction.

ment of OLT. The high scores of 88% excellent and satisfactory results have been confirmed by the experience of van Buecken and colleagues [33] and others [34,35] who have promoted wide and modified use of these techniques.

Allogenous and autogenous osteochondral transplantation, bone grafting, and ACI have been described more recently [3,36–49]. These techniques have specific indications according to the stage, location, and extent of damaged area. The age and the lifestyle of the patient also influence the specific procedure recommended.

Allografts, fresh and frozen, have been used to treat large lesions. Based on the gradual deterioration of the hyaline part of such grafts in the knee, a number of investigators have expressed their concerns with the use of allografts in the talus. Because of this concern, transplantation of osteochondral allografts is indicated only for massive osteochondral lesions, which are relatively rare in the talocrural joint [41,44].

Transplantation of free rib perichondrial flaps and periosteal flapping of osteochondral lesions in the ankle joint is still experimental, but there are a few promising clinical reports about implantation of autologous chondrocytes into OLTs [41,47]. Petersen and colleagues [47] described good early results by using the autologous chondrocyte implantation method they popularized for the treatment of OLT and chondral defects of the knee.

In contrast to the good clinical outcome, the length of the rehabilitation, high laboratory costs, and technical problems appear to be disadvantageous elements of this technique.

The type of surgical treatment also influences the exposure. Most lesions can be treated by means of arthroscopy. Many posteromedial lesions do not have to be treated by malleolar osteotomy but can be treated arthroscopically by bringing the foot into hyper–plantar flexion, although skill and experience are required [34].

Canale and Belding [9] recommended medial malleolar osteotomy when dealing with medial lesions due to their central posterior sites. In an effort to avoid osteotomy, Flick and Gould [7] suggested the use of an anteromedial approach combined with "grooving" of the anteromedial distal tibial articular surface, whereas Thompson and Loomer [50] recommended a combined anteromedial and posteromedial approach. Recently, Jakob and colleagues [43] described a technique to treat lateral defects by osteotomy of the lateral malleolus.

Bone marrow stimulation

Curettage and drilling or microfracturing

After debridement, multiple connections with the subchondral bone are created. They can be accomplished by drilling or microfracturing. The objective is to partially destroy the calcified zone that is most often present and to create multiple openings into the subchondral bone. Intraosseous blood vessels are disrupted, and the release of growth factors leads to the formation of a fibrin clot. The formation of local new blood vessels is stimulated, marrow cells are introduced in the osteochondral defect, and fibrocartilaginous tissue is formed. In the case of large defects, a cancellous bonegraft can be placed.

Preoperative considerations

Preoperatively, it has to be decided how to approach the defect. Depending on the preference of the surgeon and the location of the lesion, the approach can be from the front, from the back, or by means of a malleolar osteotomy. In the case of arthroscopic treatment, it has to be decided whether to use mechanical distraction in combination with a 2.7-mm arthroscope or to use a 4.0-mm arthroscope and treat the osteochondral defects in the anterior working area by full plantar flexion of the ankle [51]. In patients who have unlimited plantar flexion, all defects in the anterior half of the talus and lesions that are located in the anterior part of the posterior half can thus be reached and treated. The procedure is started without distraction. Introduction of the instruments is performed in the fully dorsiflexed position using the standard anteromedial and anterolateral portal [34].

Operative technique

The standard anteromedial and anterolateral approaches are created as described by van Dijk and Scholte [51]. A 4.0-mm scoop and a 4.5- or 5.5-mm shaver are introduced. When the osteochondral defect is located anteromedially, the 4.0-mm arthroscope is moved over to the anterolateral portal and the instruments are introduced through the anteromedial portal. For an anterolateral defect, the arthroscope remains in the anteromedial portal and the instruments are introduced through the anterolateral portal. When osteophytes are present, they are removed first by chisel, burr, or aggressive full-radius resector (Bone Cutter Dyonics, Smith & Nephew, Andover, Massachusetts). Synovitis located anterolaterally (in the case of an anterolateral defect) or anteromedially (in the case of an anteromedial defect) is removed first by a 4.5- or 5.5-mm full-radius resector with the ankle in the dorsiflexed position. The completeness of removal of osteophytes and synovitis is checked by bringing the ankle into plantar flexion. It should now be possible to palpate and visualize the osteochondral defect without disturbance of the synovium or overlying osteophyte. If this is not the case, then a further synovectomy is performed in the dorsiflexed position. After sufficient synovectomy, it should be possible to identify the lesion in the forced plantar flexed position by palpating the cartilage with a probe or hook. In cases of a posterior located osteochondral lesion, palpating the lesion demands a full plantar flexion. A little joint laxity helps to open up the joint. During this part of the procedure, a soft tissue distractor is applied (Fig. 5A) [51]. Not only can the lesion be palpated with a probe but it should also be possible to visualize at least the anterior part of the lesion and possibly lift it (see Fig. 5B). If possible, the 4.5- or 5.5-mm aggressive full-radius resector is now introduced into the

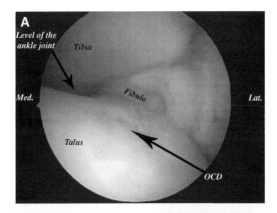

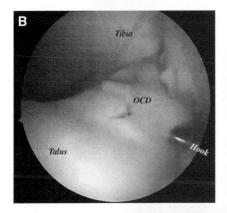

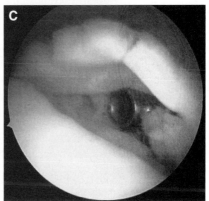

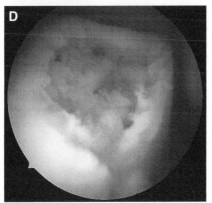

Fig. 5. Arthroscopic view of osteochondral ankle defect in left ankle. (*A*) View after distraction. The 30° scope is in the anteromedial portal, instruments introduced through the anterolateral portal. Lat., lateral; Med., medial; OCD, osteochondral defect. (*B*) The defect is lifted by a hook, showing its true size. OCD, osteochondral defect. (*C*) Excision of osteochondral defect. (*D*) Scope inserted through anterolateral portal. Direct view of defect after debridement and drilling.

defect. In doubtful cases, before introduction of the resector, it can be useful to identify the defect by introducing a spinal needle, thereby penetrating the defect area. When there is any doubt about the direction and the extent of the defect, the arthroscope is moved over to the portal opposite of the defect (the anteromedial portal in the case of an anteromedial osteochondral defect) and the completeness of the debridement is assessed. The scope is then brought back to the opposite portal and further debridement is performed by means of the aggressive full-radius resector or a small closed-cup curette (see Fig. 5C). It is important to remove all dead bone and overlying unsupported, unstable cartilage. Every step in the debridement procedure is checked by regularly switching portals. A precise and complete debridement with removal of all loose fragments can thus be performed. Introduction of the instruments and the arthroscope is performed with the ankle in the fully dorsiflexed position, thus preventing iatrogenic cartilage damage. After full debridement, the sclerotic zone is drilled by multiple drill-holes using a 2-mm burr or a 1.4-mm K-wire. A K-wire has the advantage of flexibility; a 2-mm drill can break more easily if the position of the ankle is changed during drilling. When a 2-mm drill is used, a drill sleeve is necessary to protect the tissue. Microfracturing by means of a microfracture probe offers the possibility to work "around the corner." The surgeon must make sure that the calcified area is penetrated (see Fig. 5D).

Rehabilitation

After arthroscopic debridement and drilling, patients are encouraged to make active plantar flexed and dorsiflexed ankle movements. Partial weight bearing is allowed. Full weight bearing is dependent on the size and location of the lesion. A lesion of up to 1 cm is allowed to progress to full weight bearing within 2 weeks. Larger lesions and anterior located lesions require partial weight bearing of up to 6 weeks. Running on even ground is permitted after 12 weeks. Full return to normal and sporting activities is usually possible 4 to 6 months post surgery.

Materials and methods

The authors report on two studies of a consecutive group of patients, treated by one of us (C. Niek van Dijk) for osteochondral ankle defects by means of debridement and drilling.

Between April 1988 and June 1997, 43 consecutive patients had arthroscopic treatment for an osteochondral ankle defect. Patients were seen at a minimum follow-up of 2 years; 5 were lost to follow-up. Sixteen patients had had previous surgery for the same condition. In the other 22 patients, no previous intervention had taken place (primary group).

Between October 1997 and May 1999, another group of 29 consecutive patients who had osteochondral ankle lesions was treated by means of arthroscopic debridement and drilling and prospectively followed. This group was part of a larger group of patients who had chronic ankle pain and presented at the outpatient department of the Academic Medical Center in Amsterdam, the Netherlands, and were consecutively included into a diagnostic protocol. The study was part of a prospective study design on different diagnostic strategies in patients suffering chronic ankle pain. Patients were seen for a late follow-up at 2 years after the intervention.

The outcome in both groups was assessed using the Ogilvie-Harris score, which includes pain, swelling, limping, stiffness, and activity. The patient grades each item as excellent, good, fair, or poor, with the lowest evaluation for each item determining the final score. These assessments were made before operation and at follow-up, as were the radiologic appearances using a scoring system to determine degenerative changes [9].

Results

The mean interval between the initial symptoms and surgery in the patients treated between 1988 and 1997 was 21 months (range, 6–60 months). The mean age at time of surgery was 29.3 years (range, 15–78 years) and the mean period of follow-up was 4.8 years (range, 2–11 years). Good or excellent results were found in 86% in the primary group and in 75% in the revision group. In the primary group, 9% had fair and 5% had poor results; in the revision group, 6% had fair and 19% had poor results. Only one patient in the revision group developed progression of degenerative changes that were seen at a follow-up after 10 years. In none of the other patients was there a change in radiologic grading [34].

Between 1997 and 1999, 35 osteochondral lesions were identified in 29 patients. Among these patients, 25 (86%) had a history of ankle trauma, of which 23 had a history of inversion trauma and 2 sustained an ankle fracture. Preoperative radiologic findings showed that 16 ankles had grade 0 osteoarthritic changes, 9 had grade I, and 4 had grade II. All patients returned for a 2-year follow-up.

After 2 years' follow-up, the results were excellent/good in 24 of 29 patients (83%). At the 2-year follow-up, there were no changes in grading according to the degenerative scoring scale [24].

Autologous osteochondral grafting

Single block transplants

Single block transplants involve grafting a plug from the lesser–weight bearing femoral condyle into the osteochondral defect on the talar dome. Single plug grafts result in reduced ingrowth of the fibrocartilage, although donor site morbidity may be greater because of harvesting a single, larger plug [46,48]. Similar to what is practiced in knees, the use of multiple smaller grafts (ie, mosaicplasty) is preferred, which provides a better match to the talar dome contour and surface area of the defect.

Autologous osteochondral mosaicplasty

Autologous osteochondral grafting seems to be more popular than any other "new technique" that aims to promote a hyaline-type resurfacing of the defected area. Extended experimental trials have confirmed the viability of the transplanted hyaline cartilage and fibrocartilage repair of the donor sites [52–56]. Use of multiple smaller grafts instead of one large block may help to avoid donor site morbidity. Furthermore, the congruency in the specific application of the talus may be improved. During the past 10 years, autologous osteochondral mosaicplasty became a popular treatment option for full-thickness femoral condylar lesions, and the indication had already been extended to talar lesions as early as 1992.

Preoperative considerations

An essential aspect of the procedure is insertion of the osteochondral plugs perpendicular to the recipient site. Due to the constrained configuration of the talocrural joint with its highly contoured articular surfaces, access to these lesions may be a challenge. Experience has taught that they are best approached through a miniarthrotomy, at times associated with a malleolar osteotomy. The grafts are usually obtained from the medial femoral ridge and sometimes from the lateral femoral ridge of the ipsilateral knee because these are minimal weight bearing surfaces. When the knee is precluded as a donor site, use of small (2.7- or 3.5-mm diameter) autologous grafts from the anterior talus can be considered.

Although radiographic evaluation, CT scan, or MRI may help to determine the extent of the lesion, the size of the mosaicplasty is determined after excision of the defect. Usually the patient is prepared for a mosaicplasty based on radiographic and MRI findings, but the final decision is determined during arthroscopy. Preoperatively, the patient is informed thoroughly about the possible treatments and the after-treatment. Caution should be exercised in offering the mosaicplasty to patients over age 50 years, patients who have undergone multiple previous surgeries, and patients who, regardless of age or previous surgical history, demonstrate evidence of panarticular arthritis or articular cartilage thinning.

Operative technique

Under general or spinal anesthesia, the affected lower extremity is prepared from upper thigh to toes and the thigh tourniquet is elevated to 100 mm Hg above systolic pressure. An arthroscopic survey is undertaken to further define the size, location, and surgical grade of the lesion. A final determination of the surgical treatment course is made. The ideal findings for mosaicplasty include an approximately 10-mm diameter focal osteochondral lesion, the medial or lateral dome, detached osteochondral fragments, and otherwise normal articular surfaces of the tibia and talus.

Osteoarthritis of the ankle is a contraindication; however, anterior talar and tibial osteophytes do not preclude mosaicplasty consideration. Removal is an integral part of the operation.

For medial lesions, a medial malleolar osteotomy is usually required. To ensure adequate exposure, the line of osteotomy must be made at the junction of the medial plafond. If the lesion is large and central, rotating the ankle into valgus is necessary. Use of a Steinmann pin may help to achieve eversion of the talus.

When the lesion is exposed, all diseased and suspect cartilage is removed by curette and knife blade dissection to a sharply defined rim. This vertical rim has the advantage of optimal load sharing between recipient site and transplants. The currently used mosaicplasty instruments (Mosaicplasty Complete Instrumentation, Smith & Nephew, Andover, Massachusetts) have tools for precisely measuring the intended number and diameter of grafts and the depth of the recipient holes. Size and location of the intended drill holes are edged on the base surface. The usual sizes of the drill holes in the talus are 6.5 mm and 4.5 mm in diameter. Smaller sizes such as 3.5 mm in diameter can be used to fill the dead spaces between the previously implanted grafts. These sizes allow for contouring and rotating the grafts for the desired surface confluence.

After refreshing the bony base of the defect by sharp curettage or abrasion arthroplasty, the sharp cutting edge of the appropriate-sized drill guide helps to determine an ideal filling rate of the defect. Tapping in this bevel and removing it will mark the bony base and helps to plan the filling. Primarily, the 6.5-mm size can be used to fill the defect, whereas the 4.5-mm and 3.5-mm sizes may be used to fill the remaining spaces. After completion of the recipient site preparation, osteochondral grafts are harvested from the ipsilateral knee. The primary harvest site is the medial upper part of the medial femoral condyle. As a less frequent option, the lateral supracondylar ridge can also be used through a 15- to 20-mm miniarthrotomy. By flexing the knee from 0° to 100°, three to four plugs can be obtained. When the site has been clearly identified, the proper-sized tubular chisel is located perpendicular to the articular surface and driven by hammer to the appropriate depth. Minimal graft length should be at least twice its diameter, but as a rule, plugs 25 mm in length should be taken for osteochondral defects. The grafts are procured with double-edged tubular cutting chisels that ensure the precise diameter and length of the grafts. After removal of the grafts from the chisels, there is an anticipated 0.1- to 0.2-mm expansion in their diameter, a characteristic that helps in the press-fit fixation. Each graft length is recorded. At the end of graft harvesting, a suction drain is inserted into the knee joint.

After the graft harvest, the recipient site is re-evaluated. Accumulated clot and bone debris is lavaged from the lesion base and holes. The first drill hole is made through the tubular drill guide, which also serves as the delivery tube. The depth should be 3 to 4 mm deeper than the length of the selected plug. At this stage, the first hole is enlarged by 0.1 to 0.2 mm with the use of a conic dilator. Dilation of the recipient tunnel allows easy insertion of the graft. Accordingly, drilling, dilation, and delivery are done as a combined step for each graft. After the entire set of grafts is implanted, the ankle is lavaged, observed for loose bodies, and sent through range of motion to ensure congruency of the mosaic-plasty and fluid kinematics (Fig. 6). The osteotomy is repaired with two malleolar screws inserted through predrilled holes (Fig. 7).

Lateral OLTs most frequently occur in the anterolateral surface of the dome. In most of the cases, these lesions can be reached through a vertical anterior lateral arthrotomy. By rolling the ankle through flexion and extension, perpendicular insertion of the grafts can be performed. For large posteriorly extended lesions, Gautier and colleagues [3] and Jakob and colleagues [43] promoted lateral malleolar osteotomy. Hangody and Kish [41] recommended exposure of these large defects through an anterior fibular periosteal flap containing the origin of the anterior talofibular ligament and, if necessary, the calcaneofibular ligament. The talus can then be drawn forward and rotated downward with the help of a K-wire "joy stick" driven through the body of the talus. Perfect contouring of the talar dome may represent technical challenge, but careful graft harvest and precise implantation technique can result in perfect congruency (Fig. 8).

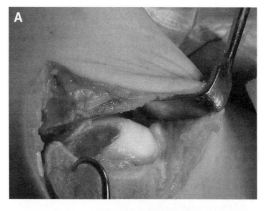

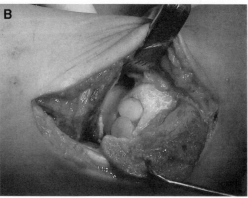

Fig. 6. Osteocontral defect on the medial talar dome. (*A*) Perpendicular approach by medial malleolar osteotomy. (*B*) Filling of the previous defect by three grafts (4.5 mm in diameter).

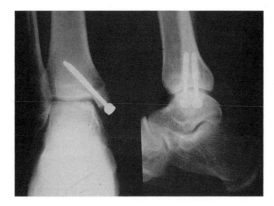

Fig. 7. Postoperative fixation of the medial malleolar osteotomy by two screws allows immediate range-of-motion exercises.

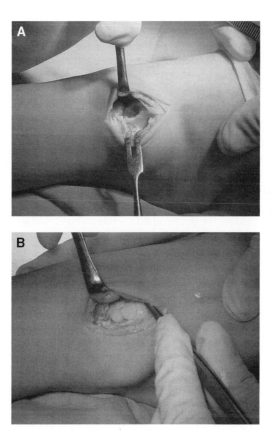

Fig. 8. Osteochondral defect on the lateral talar dome. (*A*) Perpendicular access in equine position by rolling down of the talus. (*B*) Filling of the previous defect by two grafts (6.5 mm in diameter).

An osteochondral defect that has a combined subchondral and cystic lesion can also be treated by fine technical modifications.

At the conclusion of the procedure, the tourniquet is released, bleeding is controlled, and a well-padded compression dressing is applied. The patient is observed for 24 hours to keep the extremity elevated, to administer intravenous antibiotics, and to control pain. The knee drain is removed after 24 hours.

Rehabilitation

Patients who do not undergo osteotomy are kept non–weight bearing for 3 weeks, and those who undergo medial malleolar osteotomy are kept non–weight bearing for 6 weeks. Following this period, partial weight bearing of 70 lb for 3 weeks is allowed to promote integration of the grafts. An orthosis may improve comfort. Full range-of-motion exercises are encouraged. Unprotected weight bearing is allowed at 6 weeks. Athletic activities may begin at approximately 6 months, depending on postoperative assessment.

Materials and methods

Since 1992, the authors (László Hangody and Imre Szerb) performed talar mosaicplasty in more than 80 patients. This report reviews the results of 63 consecutive patients treated between March 1992 and August 2001. All patients have been followed for a minimum of 1 year. The period of follow-up ranged from 1 to 9 years, with an average of 5.8 years.

Postoperatively, all 63 patients were assessed by clinical evaluation and scoring with the Hannover and Bandi scoring systems. Postoperative radiographs were also obtained on all patients. In addition, three-dimensional CT scans were obtained on 31 ankles and MRI on 42 ankles. Second-look arthroscopies were performed in 16 cases, and six biopsy samples were obtained postoperatively between 12 and 41 months. Biopsy specimens were analyzed histologically using the following stains: hematoxylin-eosin, picrosirius red, toluidin blue, and orcein. Histologic examination for polarization, collagen type, and enzyme histochemistry were performed. Finally, cartilage stiffness was measured during four of the second-look arthroscopies using a computerized indentometric device (Artscan 1000; Artscan Oy, Helsinki, Finland).

Results

All 63 patients were available for follow-up. The average patient age was 25.2 years (range, 16–47 years). The average follow-up for the entire series was 5.8 years (range, 1–9 years). The average-sized defect treated with mosaicplasty was 1 cm^2 (0.5–2.5 cm^2), and the average number of grafts per patient was three (range, one to seven). In most of the cases, 6.5- or 4.5-mm diameter grafts were used, whereas in one third of the cases, 3.5-mm grafts were also implanted.

All patients achieved full range of motion within 12 weeks following the surgery. No patients showed loosening or subsidence of the osteochondral graft. There were no infections or thromboembolism, but in 1 case, limited range of motion was observed due to arthrofibrosis. According to the Bandi scoring system, in 61 patients, there was no long-term morbidity at the ipsilateral knee donor site. Two patients reported slight or moderate complaints in the patellofemoral area with strenuous physical activity after the first postoperative year. According to the Hannover scoring system, 47 cases were rated excellent, 11 were rated good, 3 were rated moderate, and 2 were rated poor (these 2 were at 4 and 6 years post surgery).

By radiographic examination, the transplanted grafts were observed to incorporate into the recipient bed. All osteotomy sites (one on the lateral side and all the others on the medial side) healed without problems. Three-dimensional CT scans in 31 patients showed the recipient defects filled with a congruent surface. Most of the postoperative MRI studies showed congruency of the articular surface with a similar appearance to the surrounding articular cartilage and bone, but in 3 patients, the grafted bone showed incomplete incorporation.

The second-look arthroscopies demonstrated normal and congruent-appearing surfaces. Biopsy specimen staining showed type II specific normal articular cartilage collagen and articular cartilage proteoglycans. In five patients in whom arthroscopy was also performed postoperatively at the donor site knees, a complete fibrocartilage coverage of the defect was found to be congruent with the surrounding hyaline articular cartilage surface area. No degenerative changes in the donor areas were noted. Articular cartilage stiffness measurements showed values of 2.5 to 3.5 N compared with normal hyaline cartilage measurements of 3.5 to 4.0 N.

Autologous chondrocyte implantation/transplantation

Autologous chondrocyte implantation

ACI is defined as implantation of in vitro cultured autologous chondrocytes using a periosteal tissue cover after expansion of isolated chondrocytes. In 1965, Smith was the first person to isolate and grow chondrocytes in culture [56a]. ACI was popularized by Brittberg and colleagues [57] whose original article in the *New England Journal of Medicine* described the early results of treatment of osteochondral lesions in the knee. At 2-year follow-up, good or excellent outcomes were reported in 14 of 16 patients. Since then, ACI has been performed in over 25,000 patients. Of these cases, 95% have been in the knee, 3% in the ankle, and 2% in other joints. Based on promising early results with ACI in the knee, surgeons have begun to look at outcomes after ACI for treatment of osteochondral lesions of the talus.

Preoperative considerations

Evaluation of patients who have OLT begins with a thorough history and physical examination in addition to plain radiographs including anteroposterior, mortise, and lateral views. Weight-bearing and stress radiographs are obtained as needed. CT scans in the coronal and axial planes with sagittal reconstructions to measure the exact size of the lesion and assess the cortical outlines are used. MRI is helpful to assess quality of the overlying articular cartilage and to look for subchondral cysts but may overestimate the size of the lesion. The authors classify OLT according to a recognized CT classification system [17]. At The Southern California Orthopedic Institute, the authors (R.M. Dopirak and R.D. Ferkel) presently initially recommend nonoperative treatment for acute and chronic CT scan stage I and II lesions. When patients remain symptomatic after an extended course of conservative management, surgical intervention is recommended. For lesions that are CT scan stage III or IV, ankle arthroscopy is recommended as the initial treatment. Patients who have open growth plates receive an initial course of conservative care for grade I to III lesions and surgical intervention for grade IV lesions. Initial arthroscopic treatment of OLT typically consists of marrow-stimulating techniques.

For patients who have OLT and remain symptomatic after ankle arthroscopy with excision, curettage, and drilling, ACI is considered a viable treatment option. The defect should be focal, contained, and greater than 2 cm^2. Large lesions with subchondral cystic changes may also be treated with ACI, using the "sandwich technique." It is the authors' preference to offer ACI only to patients under age 55 years because articular chondrocytes become senescent with age [58].

Relative contraindications to ACI are bipolar lesions or diffuse degenerative joint changes. ACI is not typically offered as an initial treatment to patients who have OLT. Patients who have a large OLT and a significant cyst, however, may be candidates for ACI as the initial operative treatment because these lesions do poorly with marrow-stimulating techniques alone. Advanced osteoarthritis is an absolute contraindication to ACI. Skeletal malalignment and ligamentous instability are also absolute contraindications unless they are concomitantly corrected at the time of surgery.

Operative technique

ACI is a staged procedure. The initial surgery consists of ipsilateral knee arthroscopy for cartilage harvesting. Articular cartilage is harvested from non–weight bearing surfaces such as the intercondylar notch. Approximately 200 to 300 mg of cartilage is harvested with the use of curettes. The specimen is sent to Genzyme Tissue Repair Laboratories (Cambridge, Massachusetts) for chondrocyte isolation and proliferation. Recently, Giannini and colleagues [59] reported good results using the detached osteochondral fragment as the source of cells. Others have advocated taking a biopsy sample from a non–weight bearing part of the normal portion of the talus.

Ankle arthroscopy is also performed at the time of chondrocyte harvest to assess the size of the OLT and the status of the surrounding articular cartilage and to treat other pathology not amenable to treatment through the planned malleolar osteotomy. Arthroscopy is performed in the supine position, using a thigh holder to flex the hip to 45°. The tourniquet is inflated after exsanguination, and the foot is placed in noninvasive distraction. Standard anteromedial, anterolateral, and posterolateral portals are created. In most cases, the 2.7-mm 30° and 70° arthroscopes are used, although in some cases, a 1.9-mm arthroscope is necessary due to limited working space in the ankle. A 21-point diagnostic examination is performed to assess the OLT and to evaluate the remainder of the joint for concomitant pathology [60].

After cell preparation, the patient returns to the operating room for the second stage of the procedure, which is typically at least 4 weeks after the harvesting procedure. A medial or lateral malleolar osteotomy is necessary to provide access for the ACI procedure. The level of the osteotomy is determined intraoperatively with the assistance of fluoroscopy and preoperative scans (Fig. 9). It is essential that the osteotomy be carried medial or lateral enough to provide adequate access to the OLT [61]. Drill-holes for malleolar fixation are created before osteotomy. The osteotomy is initiated with a saw and completed with an osteotome under direct visualization. The medial malleolus is hinged inferiorly on the deltoid ligament, and the fibula is hinged posteriorly after release of the anterior inferior tibiofibular and anterior talofibular ligaments.

The malleolus is retracted to provide direct visualization of the osteochondral lesion. All pathologic fibrous and cartilaginous tissue is debrided (Fig. 10). A no. 15 blade is used to make a vertical incision at the periphery of the defect. The subchondral bone should not be penetrated during this step because this would enable marrow elements to contaminate the cultured chondrocyte population.

The periosteal graft is next obtained from the ipsilateral proximal or distal tibia. A template of the OLT is created to guide the shape and size of the periosteal resection. The periosteal graft is typically oversized by 1 to 2 mm. The graft is harvested using sharp dissection; electrosurgery is not used because of the potential for tissue necrosis. After incising the periphery of the graft with a scalpel, an elevator is used to gently separate the graft from the underlying bone. Excess soft tissue is debrided to avoid harvesting a graft of excessive thickness.

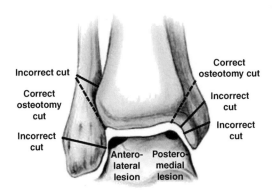

Fig. 9. ACI osteotomy. Correct malleolar osteotomy allows for adequate exposure of the OLT. (*From* Bazaz R, Ferkel RD. Treatment of osteochondral lesions of the talus with autologous chondrocyte implantation. Tech Foot Ankle Surg 2004;3(1):47; with permission.)

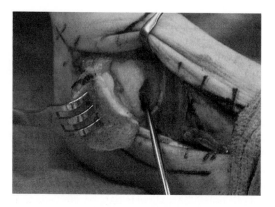

Fig. 10. Curettage of osteochondral lesion of the right medial talar dome. Note the medial malleolus has been osteotomized and is retracted inferiorly to allow exposure.

The noncambium layer is marked and the graft is stored in moist sponge to prevent graft shrinkage. The tourniquet is released and hemostasis is obtained.

With the cambium side facing toward bone, the periosteal graft is placed over the defect and secured with 5.0 or 6.0 Vicryl. The sutures are spaced 3 mm apart and the knots tied over the graft (Fig. 11). Fibrin glue is placed at the interface to help seal the graft. A small opening at the interface is left patent so that an angiocatheter can be placed into the OLT to inject the chondrocytes. Saline is injected to confirm that a watertight compartment has been created and is subsequently aspirated from the defect. It is critical to ensure that the periosteal graft does not adhere to the surface of the defect during saline removal. The cultured chondrocytes are now placed into the defect, and the insertion site is closed with the last Vicryl stitch and fibrin glue.

When there is a cystic defect in the subchondral bone, a sandwich procedure may be necessary. The cartilage of the defect is prepared as previously described.

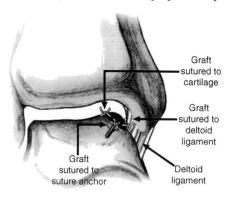

Fig. 11. Three choices to secure periosteal graft to articular cartilage: direct suture to cartilage, suture to adjacent ligament, or suture by way of minianchor into talus. (*From* Bazaz R, Ferkel RD. Treatment of osteochondral lesions of the talus with autologous chondrocyte implantation. Tech Foot Ankle Surg 2004;3(1):48; with permission.)

The cystic lesion is debrided using curettes and burr. Autogenous bone graft is obtained from iliac crest, proximal tibia, or the calcaneous. After the OLT base is drilled, the bone graft is impacted into the defect to the level of subchondral bone. In the sandwich procedure, two periosteal grafts are necessary. The first graft is placed over the bone graft with the cambium side facing toward the articular surface. This graft is secured with 6.0 Vicryl stitch and fibrin glue. The second periosteal patch is sewn over the cartilage defect with the cambium side down, and the remainder of the procedure is completed as previously described.

After completion of the ACI, the osteotomy site is reduced, and internal fixation is performed using the predrilled screw holes. The authors use three 4.0 Arbeitsgemeinschaft für Osteosynthesefragen (AO) cannulated screws for fixation of the medial malleolus. The lateral malleolar osteotomy is stabilized with a 1/3 tubular plate and two lag screws. Titanium implants are preferred in all cases to allow future MRI compatibility. The medial and lateral capsule/ligaments are repaired as needed, and routine wound closure is performed. The patient is placed in a well-padded short leg cast.

Rehabilitation

The patient remains in a well-padded short leg cast during the immediate postoperative period and is kept strictly non–weight bearing. At 2 weeks post surgery, the sutures are removed and the patient is placed in a controlled action motion walker boot. Partial weight bearing, limited to 30 lb, is permitted at this time. Gentle ankle range of motion exercises also begin at this time and are performed four to five times per day. Weight bearing is advanced based on radiographic evidence of osteotomy healing. At 6 weeks, the patient discontinues the use of the controlled action motion walker boot and transitions to a lace-up figure-eight brace that may be worn with a comfortable shoe. Formal physical therapy in a pool and on land begins at 6 weeks and consists of four phases: early phase (<8 weeks), transition phase (8–12 weeks), midphase (3–5 months), and final phase (6–12 months). Low-impact athletic activities such as cycling and skating may be started at 4 to 6 months. Repetitive impact activities such as jogging and aerobics can be resumed at 6 to 8 months. Return to hig- level sports such as basketball and football is permitted at 12 months.

Materials and methods

The authors performed ACI on 31 patients who had OLT and formally evaluated the first 11. All 11 patients failed an initial course of conservative management. All 11 patients also had prior surgery for the OLT. Four lesions involved the right ankle, and seven lesions involved the left ankle. The OLT was medial in 9 patients and lateral in 2 patients. The average size of the lesion was 13.1 mm × 20.7 mm (range, 8–28 mm). The average patient age was 33 years (range, 21–47 years). Six of the 11 patients had significant cystic subchondral extension that was treated with the sandwich procedure. No patient had a bipolar lesion. No patient had extensive degenerative changes in the joint. Second-look arthroscopy with hardware removal was performed in 10 patients. Mean follow-up of these patients was 38 months (range, 24–60 months).

Results

Ten of 11 patients reported that they were improved after the surgery; 1 patient was unchanged. At latest follow-up, outcomes were classified as good or excellent in 82% of patients (9/11). Outcomes were fair in 18% of patients (2/11). No patient had a poor outcome. The preoperative Tegner Activity Level was 1.3 ± 1.0. Postoperatively, this value improved to 4.0 ± 1.6. The American Orthopaedic Foot and Ankle Society score improved from 47.4 preoperatively to 84.3 postoperatively [62].

Second-look arthroscopy was performed in 10 patients at an average 14.2 months post surgery (range, 9–24 months). At the time of repeat arthroscopy, complete coverage of the defect was seen in all 10 patients. The cartilage at the repair site was noted to be softer than the surrounding native articular cartilage; however, it was observed that there was a correlation between firmness of the graft and total length of time from tissue implantation to second-look

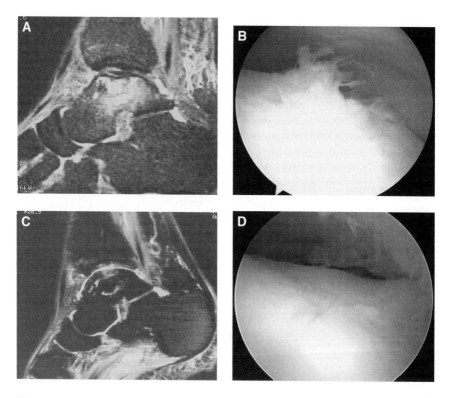

Fig. 12. Forty-seven-year-old woman who had a failed OLT surgery. (*A*) Preoperative sagittal MRI. (*B*) Preoperative arthroscopic picture of loose medial OLT. (*C*) Postoperative sagittal MRI 28 months after ACI. (*D*) Second-look arthroscopy performed 18 months after ACI.

arthroscopy. The grafts seemed to become stiffer as a function of time; the more mature grafts felt similar to the surrounding native articular cartilage on palpation (Fig. 12).

Periosteal overgrowth was noted in 2 of the 11 patients. No donor site morbidity or any complications were experienced in this study group.

Discussion

The choice of treatment for osteochondral ankle defects depends on symptomatology, duration of complaints, size of the defect, and whether it concerns a primary or secondary OLT. None of the current grading systems is sufficient to direct the choice of treatment [63].

Pure cartilage lesions, asymptomatic lesions, and low-symptomatic lesions are treated conservatively with rest, ice, temporarily reduced weight bearing, and in case of giving way, an orthosis. Consideration for surgical treatment is failure of nonoperative treatment or continuing symptoms after previous surgical treatment (secondary OLT). In recent reviews of the literature, the best current available treatment for primary osteochondral ankle defects is excison, debridement, and drilling [35,63,64]. In these reviews, osteochondral transplantation and autologous chondrocyte implantation play a minor role because results of these techniques are not yet widely published. According to the recent International Society of Arthroscopy Knee Surgery and Orthopaedic Sports Medicine–International Federation of Sports Medicine (ISAKOS—FIMS) consensus, debridement and drilling/microfracturing is the first step in the treatment of symptomatic osteochondral lesions that are too small to consider fixation [65]. In the present article, the authors report 86% favorable results at 2-years' follow-up and 83% good/excellent results at 2 to 11 years' follow-up.

Fixation with 1 or 2 lag screws is preferred in (semi)acute lesions in which the fragment is 15 mm or larger. In adolescents, refixation of an osteochondral defect should always be considered, even in fragments that are smaller than 15 mm. Large talar cystic lesions can be treated by retrograde drilling and filling the gap with a bone graft. In cases of failed primary treatment, an osteochondral transplant or cultured chondrocyte transplant can be considered.

Autologous osteochondral mosaicplasty was originally developed to treat small and medium-sized (1.0–4.0 cm^2) focal chondral and osteochondral defects of the femoral condyles and patellotrochlear surfaces. After promising early experiences in the knee, the indication has been extended to OLTs. A perpendicular approach to the defect often requires a relatively aggressive approach such as medial malleolar osteotomy. On the lateral side, an osteotomy can usually be avoided. Central and caput tali lesions can be treated by demanding special approaches. According to Christel and colleagues [37], talar mosaicplasty represents a more difficult technique than knee application. They also reported less favorable clinical outcomes in the ankle than in the knee. Other investigators such as Assenmacher and colleagues [36], Gautier and colleagues

[3], and Imhoff and colleagues [42] reported promising clinical outcomes similar to the authors' reports. They also recommended this technique in cases of previous failed procedures. Recently, several other reports confirmed the advantageous initial clinical experiences with the talar mosaicplasty technique [38,45,48,49].

The treatment technique involves only one operation but two incisions, with one at the ankle and one at the knee. The donor area for the graft harvest is the ipsilateral knee, the lesser–weight bearing edges of the femoral condyles at the level of the patellofemoral joint. As has been demonstrated in other publications, these donor site holes eventually fill with cancellous bone and are covered by fibrocartilage, which is acceptable support for the stresses of this relatively lesser–weight bearing portion of the patellofemoral joint [1,21,26]. Although hyaline cartilage of the donor area located in the knee is certainly different from the talar hyaline cartilage, there is no evidence to date that this represents a negative influence in the long-term results.

Newer techniques such as ACI offer a promising treatment alternative, but long-term data are lacking. ACI has been shown to yield favorable long-term results in the knee [66], but these findings cannot be directly extrapolated to OLT. To date, only short-term data are available on the treatment of OLT with ACI. The authors noted an improvement in 10 of 11 patients at a mean follow-up of 36 months. Other investigators have similarly reported favorable results at short-term follow-up [47,67,68]. Long-term studies, however, are needed to evaluate the efficacy of this technique.

In addition, the biologic and mechanical properties of the regenerative tissue after ACI remain undefined. Histologic data are needed to determine whether the repair tissue formed in the talus is the same hyaline-like tissue that is formed in the knee. Incomplete healing of subchondral cysts after ACI was noted in some of the authors' patients; although this did not seem to adversely influence clinical outcomes at short-term follow-up, the long-term effect of these cysts is unknown.

Until further data are available, the authors cannot advocate ACI as an initial treatment option for most cases of OLT. In patients who have failed prior surgical treatment for OLT and in patients who have large subchondral bone defects, however, the short-term data suggest that ACI can provide good results.

Outside of the United States, newer techniques have recently been developed using scaffolds implanted with cultured chondrocytes to treat OLT [69–71]. The membrane/matrix ACI (MACI) technique makes use of a bovine collagen membrane that serves as the scaffold for implanted chondrocytes. The chondrocyte-populated membrane may be implanted directly into the OLT arthroscopically or by way of a miniarthrotomy, obviating the need for a malleolar osteotomy. Periosteal graft harvest is not necessary with the MACI technique because the membrane may be directly sutured into place or sealed with fibrin glue. Ronga and colleagues [70] and Guillen and colleagues [71] reported on outcomes after MACI for the treatment of OLT; short-term results in these small cohorts of patients are encouraging.

Table 1
Guideline for treatment of osteochondral talar lesions

Lesion	Treatment
Type 1: asymptomatic lesions, low-symptomatic lesions	Conservative
Type 2: symptomatic lesions ≤10 mm	Debridement and drilling/microfracturing
Type 3: symptomatic lesions 11–14 mm	Consider debridement and drilling, fixation, an osteochondral graft, or ACI
Type 4: symptomatic lesions ≥15 mm	Consider fixation, graft, or ACI
Type 5: large talar cystic lesions	Consider retrograde drilling ± bone transplant, or ACI with sandwich procedure
Type 6: secondary lesions	Consider osteochondral transplant

For types 4 through 6, debridement and bone marrow stimulation can always be considered a treatment option.

Hyalograft C is another biocompatible scaffold for chondrocyte implantation. This graft can be implanted arthroscopically without the need for a malleolar osteotomy for exposure or a periosteal flap for fixation [72]. Giannini and colleagues [73] performed arthroscopic ACI in 30 patients using Hyalograft C as the scaffold, with good short-term results. At the time of writing this manuscript, these scaffolds have not been approved for use in the United States, although they hold great promise for the treatment of OLT in the future.

Because none of the current grading systems is sufficient to direct the choice of treatment [64], the authors propose that, as a guideline, the size of the lesion be used as main indicator for treatment (Table 1).

Summary

An OLT often causes pain, recurrent synovitis, and obstruction from loose bodies. It is a possible precursor of ankle osteoarthritis due to altered joint mechanics and recurrent synovitis. Current diagnostic strategies usually include MRI or CT. Recent research has shown that MRI and CT have the same diagnostic accuracy in the diagnosis of an OLT. For preoperative planning, a CT scan gives more precise information.

Arthroscopic procedures like debridement and drilling, by nature of their minimally invasive approach, have great advantage in treating typical defects of up to 1 cm in diameter. For larger osteochondral defects, the optimal treatment result is the long-term replacement and integration of type-specific hyaline cartilage. In principle, mosaicplasty autologous osteochondral transplantation fills these criteria. The early and medium-term encouraging results, complete with confirmatory radiographs and histology, hold promise for this procedure in lasting relief of symptoms and prevention of ankle arthrosis. ACI is a relatively new but promising treatment. Choice of treatment is thwarted by the fact that none of the current grading systems is dually related to current treatment options. Table 1 presents a guideline for treatment that is primarily based on the size of the lesion. Because of the many different operative treatment strategies that have reported satisfactory results and because of the fact that there are only few comparative studies, there is a need for randomized, prospective studies to define and validate available treatment.

Acknowledgments

Peter de Leeuw is gratefully acknowledged for recording the images in Fig. 5A through 5D.

References

[1] DeBerardino TM, Arciero RA, Taylor DC. Arthroscopic treatment of soft tissue impingement of the ankle in athletes. Arthroscopy 1997;13(4):492–8.

[2] McCullough CJ, Venugopal V. Osteochondritis dissecans of the talus: the natural history. Clin Orthop Relat Res 1979;144:264–8.

[3] Gautier E, Jung M, Mainil-Varlet P, et al. Articular surface repair in the talus using autogenous osteochondral plug transplantation. A preliminary report. Int Cartilage Rep Soc Newslett 1999; 1:19–20.

[3a] Monro A. Microgeologie. Berlin: Th. Billroth, 1856:236.

[4] Paget J. On the production of the loose bodies in joints. St. Bartholomew's Hospital Rep 1870; 6:1.

[4a] König F. Über freie Körper in den Gelenken. [On the presence of loose bodies in joints]. Deutsche Zeitschrift für Chirurgie 1887–1888;27:90–109.

[5] Rendu A. Fracture intra-articulair parcellaire de la poulie astragalienne. [Fragmented intra-articular fractures of the talar dome]. Lyon Med 1932;150:220–2.

[6] Davidson AM, Steele HD, MacKenzie DA, et al. A review of twenty-one cases of transchondral fracture of the talus. J Trauma 1967;7(3):378–415.

[7] Flick AB, Gould N. Osteochondritis dissecans of the talus (transchondral fractures of the talus): a review of the literature and a new surgical approach for medial dome lesions. Foot Ankle 1985;5(4):165–85.

[8] Nash WC, Baker CL. Transchondral talar dome fractures: not just a sprained ankle. South Med J 1984;77(5):560–4.

[9] Canale ST, Belding RH. Osteochondral lesions of the talus. J Bone Joint Surg Am 1980;62(1): 97–102.

[10] Katcherian D. Soft-tissue injuries of the ankle. In: Lufter LD, Mizel MS, Pfeffer GB, editors. Orthopaedic knowledge update: foot and ankle. Rosemont (IL): American Academy of Orthopaedic Surgeons; 1994. p. 241–53.

[11] Garrick JG. The frequency of injury, mechanism of injury, and epidemiology of ankle sprains. Am J Sports Med 1977;5(6):241–2.

[12] Bosien WR, Staples OS, Russel SW. Residual disability following acute ankle sprains. J Bone Joint Surg Am 1955;37(6):1237–43.

[13] Van Dijk CN. On diagnostic strategies in patients with severe ankle sprain [dissertation]. Amsterdam, the Netherlands: University of Amsterdam; 1994.

[14] Lippert MJ, Hawe W, Bernett P. Surgical therapy of fibular capsule-ligament rupture. Sportverletz Sportschaden 1989;3(1):6–13 [in German].

[15] Berndt AL, Harty M. Transchondral fractures (osteochondritis dissecans) of the talus. J Bone Joint Surg Am 1959;41:988–1020.

[16] Anderson IF, Crichton KJ, Grattan-Smith T, et al. Osteochondral fractures of the dome of the talus. J Bone Joint Surg Am 1989;71(8):1143–52.

[17] Ferkel RD, Sgaglione NA, Del Pizzo W. Arthroscopic treatment of osteochondral lesions of the talus: techniques and results. Orthop Trans 1990;14:172.

[18] Frank A, Cohen P, Beaufils P, et al. Arthroscopic treatment of osteochondral lesions of the talar dome. Arthroscopy 1989;5(1):57–61.

[19] Hepple S, Winson IG, Glew D. Osteochondral lesions of the talus: a revised classification. Foot Ankle Int 1999;20(12):789–93.

[20] Anderson DV, Lyne ED. Osteochondritis dissecans of the talus: case report on two family members. J Pediatr Orthop 1984;4(3):356–7.

[21] Erban WK, Kolberg K. Simultaneous mirror image osteochondrosis dissecans in identical twins. Rofo 1981;135(3):357 [in German].

[22] Woods K, Harris I. Osteochondritis dissecans of the talus in identical twins. J Bone Joint Surg Br 1995;77(2):331.

[23] Frenkel SR, Di Cesare PE. Degradation and repair of articular cartilage. Front Biosci 1999; 15(4):D671–85.

[24] Verhagen RA, Maas M, Dijkgraaf MG, et al. Prospective study on diagnostic strategies in osteochondral lesions of the talus. Is MRI superior to helical CT? J Bone Joint Surg Br 2005; 87(1):41–6.

[25] Alexander AH, Lichtman DM. Surgical treatment of transchondral talar-dome fractures (osteochondritis dissecans). Long-term follow-up. J Bone Joint Surg Am 1980;62(4):646–52.

[26] Baker Jr CL, Parisien JS. Arthroscopic surgery in osteocartilaginous lesions of the ankle. In: McGinty JB, editor. Operative arthroscopy. 2nd edition. Philadelphia: Lippincott–Raven; 1996. p. 1157–72.

[27] Bryant III DD, Siegel MG. Osteochondritis dissecans of the talus: a new technique for arthroscopic drilling. Arthroscopy 1993;9(2):238–41.

[28] Guhl JF, Johnson RP, Stone JW. The impact of arthroscopy on osteochondritis dissecans. In: McGinty JB, editor. Operative arthroscopy. 2nd edition. Philadelphia: Lippincott–Raven; 1996.

[29] Kumai T, Takakura Y, Tanaka Y, et al. Cortical bone peg fixation for osteochondral lesions of the talus. Presented at the 29th Annual Meeting of the American Orthopaedic Foot and Ankle Society. Anaheim, California, February 7, 1999.

[30] Parisien JS. Arthroscopic treatment of osteochondral lesions of the talus. Am J Sports Med 1986;14(3):211–7.

[31] Shea MP, Manoli II A. Osteochondral lesions of the talar dome. Foot Ankle 1993;14(1):48–55.

[32] Thermann H. Treatment of osteochondritis dissecans of the talus: a long term follow-up. Sports Med Arthrosc Rev 1993;2:284–8.

[33] Van Buecken K, Barrack RL, Alexander AH, et al. Arthroscopic treatment of transchondral talar dome fractures. Am J Sports Med 1989;17(3):350–6.

[34] Schuman L, Struijs PAA, van Dijk CN. Arthroscopic treatment for osteochondral defects of the talus. Results at follow-up at 2 to 11 years. J Bone Joint Surg Br 2002;84(3):364–8.

[35] Tol JL, Struijs PAA, Bossuyt PM, et al. Treatment strategies in osteochondral defects of the talar dome: a systematic review. Foot Ankle Int 2000;21(2):119–26.

[36] Assenmacher JA, Kelikian AS, Gottlob C, et al. Arthroscopically assisted autologous osteochondral transplantation for osteochondral lesions of the talar dome: an MRI and clinical follow-up study. Foot Ankle Int 2001;22(7):544–51.

[37] Christel P, Versier G, Landreau Ph, et al. Les greffes osteo-chondrales selon la technique de la mosaiplasty. [Osteochondral grafts according to the mosaicplasty technique]. Maitrise Orthopedique 1998;76:1–13.

[38] Gobbi A, Mahajan S, Tuy B. Osteochondral lesions of the talus. A four year follow-up study in athletes. Presented at the 4th Symposium of the International Cartilage Repair Society. Toronto, Canada, June 15–18, 2002.

[39] Hangody L, Kish G, Kárpáti Z, et al. Treatment of osteochondritis dissecans of the talus: use of the mosaicplasty technique—preliminary report. Foot Ankle Int 1997;18(10):628–34.

[40] Hangody L, Kish G, Modis L, et al. Mosaicplasty for the treatment of osteochondritis dissecans of the talus—two to seven year results in 36 patients. Foot Ankle Int 2001;22(7):552–8.

[41] Hangody L, Kish G. Surgical treatment of osteochondritis dissecans of the talus. In: Duparc, editor. European textbook on surgical techniques in orthopaedics and traumatology. Editions Scientifiques et Medicales Elsevier; 2000. p. 1–5.

[42] Imhoff AB, Oettl GM, Burkart A, et al. Extended indication for osteochondral autografts in different joints. Presented at the 2nd Symposium of the International Cartilage Repair Society. Boston, November 16–18, 1998.

[43] Jakob RP, Mainil-Varlet P, Saager C, et al. Mosaicplasty in cartilaginous lesions over 4 cm^2 and indications outside the knee. Cartilage repair. Presented at the 2nd Fribourg International Symposium, Fribourg, Switzerland, October 29–31, 1997.

[44] Kim CW, Bugbee W. Ankle osteochondral allografts. Presented at the 29th Annual Meeting of the American Orthopaedic Foot and Ankle Society. Anaheim, California, February 7, 1999.

[45] Kolker D, Wilson MG. Autologous osteochondral grafting for cartilage defects of the talar dome. Presented at the 4th Symposium of the International Cartilage Repair Society. Toronto, Canada, June 15–18, 2002.

[46] Martin TL, Wilson MG, Robledo J. Early results of autologous bone grafting for large talar osteochondritis dissecans lesions. Presented at the 29th Annual Meeting of the American Orthopaedic Foot and Ankle Society. Anaheim, California, February 7, 1999.

[47] Petersen L, Brittberg M, Lindahl A. Autologous chondrocyte transplantation of the ankle. Foot Ankle Clin 2003;8(2):291–303.

[48] Speck M, Schweinfurt M, Boerner T. Osteochondral autograft transplantation for traumatic and degenerative lesions of the talus. Presented at the 4th Symposium of the International Cartilage Repair Society. Toronto, Canada, June 15–18, 2002.

[49] Schaefer DB, Martin I, Dick W. Mosaicplasty for the treatment of osteochondral lesions of the talus. Presented at the 4th Symposium of the International Cartilage Repair Society. Toronto, Canada, June 15–18, 2002.

[50] Thompson JP, Loomer RL. Osteochondral lesions of the talus in a sports medicine clinic. A new radiographic technique and surgical approach. Am J Sports Med 1984;12(6):460–3.

[51] Van Dijk CN, Scholte D. Arthroscopy of the ankle joint. Arthroscopy 1997;13(1):90–6.

[52] Bodó G, Hangody L, Szabó Zs, et al. Arthroscopic autologous osteochondral mosaicplasty for the treatment of subchondral cystic lesion in the medial femoral condyle in a horse. Acta Vet Hung 2000;48(3):343–54.

[53] Bodó G, Kaposi AD, Hangody L, et al. The surgical technique and the age of the horse both influence the outcome of mosaicplasty in a cadaver equine stifle model. Acta Vet Hung 2001;49(1):111–6.

[54] Hangody L, Kárpáti Z. A new surgical treatment of localised cartilaginous defects of the knee. Hung J Orthop Trauma 1994;37:237–43.

[55] Hangody L, Feczkó P, Bartha L, et al. Mosaicplasty for the treatment of articular defects of the knee and ankle. Clin Orthop Relat Res 2001;391(Suppl):S328–36.

[56] Hangody L, Kish G, Kárpáti Z, et al. Autogenous osteochondral graft technique for replacing knee cartilage defects in dogs. Orthop Int 1997;5(3):175–81.

[56a] Smith AV. Survival of frozen chondrocytes isolated from cartilage of adult mammals. Nature 1965;205:782–4.

[57] Brittberg M, Lindahl A, Nilsson A, et al. Treatment of deep cartilage defects in the knee with autologous chondrocyte transplantation. N Engl J Med 1994;331(14):889–95.

[58] Buckwalter JA. Articular cartilage injuries. Clin Orthop Rel Res 2002;402:21–37.

[59] Giannini S, Buda R, Grigolo B, et al. The detached osteochondral fragment as a source of cells for autologous chondrocyte implantation (ACI) in the ankle joint. Osteoarth Cartilage 2005;13(7):601–7.

[60] Ferkel RD. Arthroscopic surgery: the foot and ankle. Philadelphia: Lippincott-Raven; 1996.

[61] Bazaz R, Ferkel RD. Treatment of osteochondral lesions of the talus with autologous chondrocyte implantation. Tech Foot Ankle Surg 2004;3(1):45–52.

[62] Nam EK, Ferkel RD, Applegate GR. Autologous chondrocyte implantation of the ankle: two to five year follow-up. Presented at Specialty Day, American Orthopaedic Society for Sports Medicine. San Francisco, 2004.

[63] Verhagen RA, Struijs PAA, Bossuyt PM, et al. Systematic review of treatment strategies for osteochondral defects of the talar dome. Foot Ankle Clin 2003;8(2):233–42.

[64] Struijs PA, Tol JL, Bossuyt PM, et al. Treatment strategies in osteochondral lesions of the talus. Review of the literature. Orthopade 2001;30(1):28–36 [in German].

[65] Chan KM, Karlsson I. Ankle instability. Chronic Injury—Management of Osteochondral defect. Presented at the 2005 biennial ISAKOS Congress.

[66] Peterson L, Brittberg M, Kiviranta I, et al. Autologous chondrocyte transplantation. Biomechanics and long-term durability. Am J Sports Med 2002;30(1):2–12.

[67] Giannini S, Buda R, Grigolo B, et al. Autologous chondrocyte transplantation in osteochondral lesions of the ankle joint. Foot Ankle Int 2001;22(6):513–7.

[68] Koulalis D, Schultz W, Heyden M. Autologous chondrocyte transplantation for osteochondritis dissecans of the talus. Clin Orthop Rel Res 2002;395:186–92.

[69] Basad E, Sturz H, Steinmeyer J. Treatment of chondral defects by matrix-guided autologous chondrocyte implantation (MACI). In: Hendrich C, Nöth U, Eulert J, editors. Cartilage surgery and future perspectives. Berlin: Springer-Verlag; 2003. p. 49–56.

[70] Ronga M, Grassi FA, Montoli C, et al. Treatment of deep cartilage defects of the ankle with matrix-induced autologous chondrocyte implantation (MACI). Foot Ankle Surg 2005;11: 29–33.

[71] Guillen P, Abelow S, Jaen TF. Treatment of osteochondral lesions of the talus with MACI. Presented at the 23rd AANA Fall Course. December 2004.

[72] Marcacci M, Berruto M, Brocchetta D, et al. Articular cartilage engineering with Hyalograft C: 3-year clinical results. Clin Orthop Rel Res 2005;435:96–105.

[73] Giannini S, Buda R, Faldini C, et al. Surgical treatment of osteochondral lesions of the talus in young active patients. J Bone Joint Surg Am 2005;87(Suppl 2):28–41.

ELSEVIER
SAUNDERS

Foot Ankle Clin N Am
11 (2006) 361–368

FOOT AND
ANKLE CLINICS

Arthroscopic Ankle Arthrodesis

James W. Stone, MD

2901 W. Kinnickinnic River Parkway, Suite 102, Milwaukee, WI 53215, USA

Surgical options are limited for the patient who has symptomatic severe ankle joint degeneration that is unresponsive to nonoperative treatment. Arthrodesis of the tibiotalar joint is a procedure that can produce a pain-free ankle that can withstand the rigors of daily life, even in a young, high-demand, working individual. The procedure has a long orthopedic history, with multiple options available to achieve the goal of ankle fusion. Open approaches to the ankle joint have traditionally been used, with methods including flat-cut osteotomies of the tibia and talus, sliding grafts, and in situ fusion. Methods of fixation have included cast immobilization, screws, plates, and external fixators. There is a high incidence of complications, however, with the various methods of open ankle arthrodesis. These complications include nonunion, delayed union, malunion, infection, wound necrosis, subtalar joint degeneration, neurovascular injury, and reflex sympathetic dystrophy [1]. Minimally invasive orthopedic techniques have been applied to ankle arthrodesis, and arthroscopic ankle fusion has been shown to be an effective technique to achieve tibiotalar arthrodesis, with high rates of fusion and low rates of complication [2].

Indications

The indications for arthroscopic ankle arthrodesis are the same as for open ankle arthrodesis [3]. The primary indication for the procedure is pain resulting from joint degeneration that cannot be controlled with nonoperative measures such as medications (including nonsteroidal anti-inflammatory drugs, glucosamine, and non-narcotic analgesics), corticosteroid injections, orthotics, braces, and shoe modifications. Other indications for fusion include joint deformity or

---

E-mail address: bonanza83b@aol.com

1083-7515/06/$ – see front matter © 2006 Elsevier Inc. All rights reserved.
doi:10.1016/j.fcl.2006.03.007

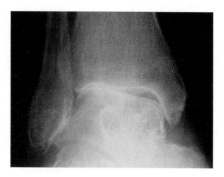

Fig. 1. Anteroposterior radiograph showing complete loss of joint space over lateral ankle joint.

instability. The etiology of ankle joint degeneration is most commonly post traumatic because primary osteoarthritis is less common in the ankle joint than in the other weight bearing joints of the lower extremity, including the hip and the knee (Fig. 1). Other less common causes of joint degeneration that may require arthrodesis include rheumatoid arthritis, crystalline arthritis, or other inflammatory arthropathy; postinfectious arthritis; osteochondral lesions of the talar dome; and avascular necrosis.

The primary contraindication for arthroscopic ankle arthrodesis is fixed varus or valgus malalignment that precludes achievement of neutral ankle position without significant bone resection from the talus or tibia.

Procedure

Arthroscopic ankle arthrodesis can be performed in the hospital or the outpatient surgery setting under general or spinal anesthetic. A tourniquet is applied to the thigh but is generally not required for this procedure. The patient is placed supine on the operating table and the ipsilateral hip and knee are flexed and supported by a well-padded leg holder (Fig. 2). The leg holder should have a long thigh component and short leg component so that when distraction force is applied to the extremity, pressure in the popliteal space is avoided. This position allows the leg to hang freely, facilitating skin preparation and draping. The noninvasive joint distractor is applied after draping. The distractor consists of a sterile strap that is locked over the heel and the midfoot. The strap is attached to a sterile post fixed to the side rail of the table, and distraction force is applied in a controlled fashion using a strip of two-sided Velcro (Fig. 3). This setup provides several advantages: the foot and ankle rest in a plantigrade position, and the ankle can be manipulated intraoperatively in dorsiflexion and plantarflexion. In addition, the position allows easy access to anterior and posterior portals. Joint distraction affords easier joint opening without the need for an assistant to provide the force on an intermittent and inconsistent basis. Other methods of distraction, including a sterile strap wrapped around the body of the surgeon

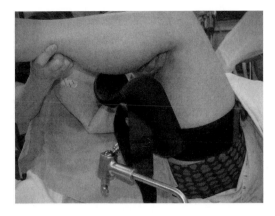

Fig. 2. Thigh holder with long thigh segment and short leg segment used for countertraction.

who then provides traction by leaning backward while operating or the patient's leg hanging dependent and weights applied to the joint, are alternatives to strap distraction.

The anteromedial portal is established first, taking advantage of the notch of Hardy, a consistent but variably sized indentation in the anterior tibia at this level that generally allows easier manipulation of the arthoscope from the medial side (Fig. 4). A hypodermic needle is used to localize appropriate position, immediately adjacent to the medial border of the anterior tibial tendon at the level

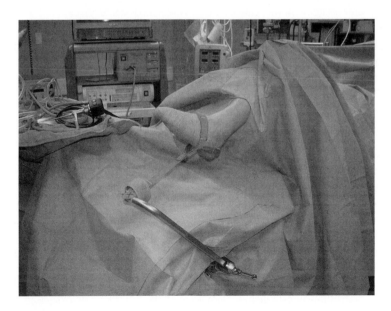

Fig. 3. Arthroscopic setup with noninvasive ankle distractor applied to the prepped and draped lower extremity.

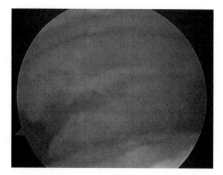

Fig. 4. Initial arthroscopic view showing complete articular cartilage loss over lateral tibiotalar joint.

of the joint line. The portal should be placed at the level at which the needle most easily traverses the joint space. The presence of a large anterior tibial osteophyte in the degenerative ankle may initially make introduction of the cannula difficult.

It is important to use correct portal establishment technique to avoid injury to superficial nerves. In each case, only the skin should be incised with the scalpel blade, being careful not to cut into the subcutaneous tissues, which are then spread with a mosquito clamp to the level of the joint capsule. The capsule is then penetrated with a blunt obturator. Each portal should also be made slightly larger than the diameter of the required cannulas and shaver blades to avoid trauma to the soft tissues during instrument passage. This technique decreases the likelihood of wound healing problems and sinus tract formation.

The anterolateral portal can be established next while visualizing from the anteromedial portal. Again, a hypodermic needle guides the appropriate level for portal placement, adjacent to the lateral border of the peroneus tertius tendon. Injury to branches of the superficial peroneal nerve, which are sometimes visible beneath the skin, is avoided using the proper portal establishment technique as described previously.

The location for the posterolateral portal is determined by placing the hypodermic needle immediately adjacent to the lateral border of the Achilles tendon and 1 to 2 cm distal to the level of the anterior portals. The needle is angled upward slightly to accommodate the curvature of the posterior talus, and entry into the joint is confirmed immediately beneath the posterior syndesmotic ligaments. Inflow is initially placed using the posterior cannula but can be varied intraoperatively so that other instruments can be placed posterior if necessary. Use of a separate inflow cannula facilitates gravity inflow. Alternatively, an arthroscopic fluid pump can be used.

It may be necessary to perform an anterior joint synovectomy to achieve initial visualization, and care must be exercised to avoid soft tissue injury anteriorly. The shaver blade should be pointed only toward the surfaces of the talus and tibia until visualization is established—not toward the anterior soft tissues in which case inadvertent capsular penetration can cause neurovascular injury. These joints usually have a large anterior tibial osteophyte that must be debrided to achieve

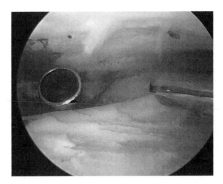

Fig. 5. Removal of remaining articular cartilage using arthroscopic shaver.

adequate joint visualization and to allow adequate apposition of the two joint surfaces at the conclusion of the case.

Any remaining articular cartilage must then be removed from the joint surfaces. Areas of thicker articular cartilage are most easily removed using a motorized shaver (Fig. 5). Alternatively, a small, curved osteotome may be introduced to scrape off articular cartilage, and the large pieces are removed with shaver or loose body forceps. The articular cartilage should be removed from the entire surface of the talus and tibia in addition to the medial and lateral gutters. A curette can be introduced into each gutter to clean it out with an up-and-down motion, and the shaver can be used to remove any remaining cartilage.

When it is difficult to reach the posterior surface of the talus or tibia, angled curettes introduced from anterior or from the posterolateral portal can facilitate debridement (Fig. 6). After removal of the articular cartilage, the next step is to remove a thin, 1- to 2-mm, layer of the subchondral bone to the level of viable bleeding bone. It is important during this process to maintain the normal bone contours of the talus and tibia so as to maximize the surface area of apposition for potential bone fusion. The amount of joint space is often adequate to introduce a large (5.5-mm) round abrader for the more anterior portions of the joint. A

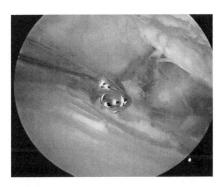

Fig. 6. Removal of posterior articular cartilage using angle curette.

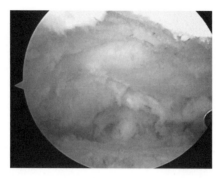

Fig. 7. Articular surfaces denuded of articular cartilage and abraded to the level of viable bleeding subchondral bone.

smaller 4-mm abrader may be necessary to reach the more posterior aspect of the joint, and it may also be introduced from posterior if required.

The adequacy of the abrasion of the bony surface can be assessed by decreasing the inflow pressure and assessing the amount of bleeding from the talus and tibia. Further abrasion should be performed on any area that is noted to remain avascular. In addition, some investigators have suggested that small "spot welds" be placed using the smaller of the two abraders introduced more deeply into the bone at intervals across the surface of the talar dome and tibial plafond (Fig. 7).

There are several options for internal fixation of the ankle arthrodesis. The author recommends using 6.5-mm self-drilling, self-tapping, cannulated screws. Crossed screws can be used—one placed from the medial side and one from the lateral side. The lateral screw can traverse the fibula and then engage the talus. Both screws are angled to place the screw threads into the talar neck if possible (Fig. 8). Alternatively, two medial screws can be placed parallel and directed into the talar neck. The crossed screw configuration provides greater rigidity, but parallel medial screw placement allows compression during weight bearing. Some investigators have advocated the use of a third screw placed anterior to posterior or posterior to anterior to increase the rigidity of the fixation; however, excellent rates have been reported with two-screw fixation.

The author generally places the guide pins under arthroscopic visualization to ensure that they are angled properly to engage the talus. After the pins are noted to be in good position, they are withdrawn to just beneath the surface of the bone. The leg is removed from the holder and placed flat on the operating table. The fluoroscope is brought in to confirm adequate position of the pins. The assistant holds the ankle in proper position for fusion: neutral dorsiflexion and slight hindfoot valgus, with compression across the joint. Varus position of the hindfoot must be avoided. When crossed pins are used, one pin is advanced first. Good position is confirmed using anteroposterior and lateral fluoroscopic views, and the screw is advanced and tightened into position to afford compression across the joint. The other pin is advanced, and the appropriate length screw is placed.

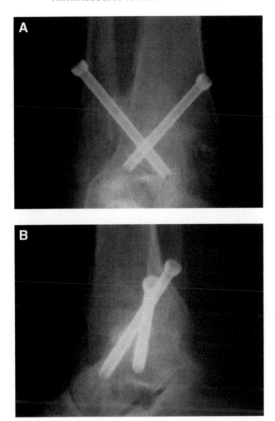

Fig. 8. (*A*) Anteroposterior and (*B*) lateral postoperative radiographs showing crossed transmalleolar screw fixation of arthoscopic ankle arthrodesis.

After screw placement, the ankle should be visualized using anteroposterior, lateral, and oblique fluoroscopic views to confirm good position, and in particular to be certain that the subtalar joint has not been penetrated. The wounds are closed with simple sutures. A bulky compressive dressing and posterior plaster splint are applied.

The sutures are removed 1 week postoperative. The ankle is placed into a short leg cast or a removable walking boot that is worn full-time except for washing. Weight bearing may be advanced as tolerated. The boot is worn until radiographic fusion is noted, usually 9 to 12 weeks postoperative.

Results

Glick and colleagues [4] reported on the first significant series of patients undergoing arthroscopic ankle arthrodesis, presenting their average 8-year long-term follow-up in 1996. Of 34 procedures performed, there was only one nonunion (fusion rate of 97%), and good or excellent results were obtained in 86%. Myerson and Quill [5] compared 17 patients undergoing arthroscopic arthrodesis with 16 patients undergoing open arthrodesis with malleolar osteotomy. These investigators found a mean time to fusion of 8.7 weeks for the arthroscopic group compared with 14.5 weeks for the open group, with similar rates of fusion. O'Brien and colleauges [6] compared a group of 19 arthroscopic fusions to 17 open fusions using flat-cut osteotomies and found that the two techniques had comparable fusion rates but that the arthroscopic procedure had less morbidity, shorter operative times, shorter tourniquet times, less blood loss, and shorter hospital stays. Review of multiple reports suggests that in patients who have minimal deformity, arthroscopic ankle arthrodesis is a reliable method for achieving ankle fusion, with fusion times of 8 to 12 weeks and an expected non-union rate of 5% to 10%. Patients who have avascular necrosis of the talus probably have a high rate of nonunion whether arthroscopic or open techniques are used [7–12].

References

[1] Morgan CD, Henke JA, Bailey RW, et al. Long-term results of tibiotalar arthrodesis. J Bone Joint Surg Am 1985;67:546–50.
[2] Crosby LA, Yee TC, Formanek TC, et al. Complications following arthroscopic ankle arthrodesis. Foot Ankle Int 1996;17:340–2.
[3] Fitzgibbons TC. Arthroscopic ankle debridement and fusion: indications, techniques, and results. Instr Course Lect 1999;48:243–8.
[4] Glick JM, Morgan CD, Myerson MS, et al. Ankle arthrodesis using an arthroscopic method: long-term follow-up of 34 cases. Arthroscopy 1996;12:428–34.
[5] Myerson MS, Quill G. Ankle arthrodesis: a comparison of an arthroscopic and an open method of treatment. Clin Orthop 1991;268:84–95.
[6] O'Brien TS, Hart TS, Shereff MJ, et al. Open versus arthroscopic ankle arthrodesis: a comparative study. Foot Ankle Int 1999;20:368–74.
[7] Cameron SE, Ullrich P. Arthroscopic arthrodesis of the ankle joint. Arthroscopy 2000;16:21–6.
[8] Corso SJ, Zimmer TJ. Technique and clinical evaluation of arthroscopic ankle arthrodesis. Arthroscopy 1995;11:585–90.
[9] Dent CM, Patil M, Fairclough JA. Arthroscopic ankle arthrodesis. J Bone Joint Surg Br 1993; 75:830–2.
[10] Glick JM, Ferkel RD. Arthroscopic ankle arthrodesis. In: Ferkel RD, editor. Arthroscopic surgery: the foot and ankle. Philadelphia: Lippincott-Raven; 1996. p. 215–29.
[11] Ogilvie-Harris DJ, Lieberman I, Fitsialos D. Arthroscopically assisted arthrodesis for osteoarthrotic ankles. J Bone Joint Surg Am 1993;75:1167–74.
[12] Zvijac JE, Lemak L, Schurhoff MR, et al. Analysis of arthroscopically assisted ankle arthrodesis. Arthroscopy 2002;18:70–5.

ELSEVIER
SAUNDERS

Foot Ankle Clin N Am
11 (2006) 369–390

FOOT AND
ANKLE CLINICS

Arthroscopy of the Posterior Subtalar Joint

Lijkele Beimers, MD[a],*, Carol Frey, MD[b],
C. Niek van Dijk, MD, PhD[a]

[a]*Department of Orthopaedic Surgery, Academic Medical Center, PO Box 22660 1100 DD Amsterdam,
The Netherlands*
[b]*Department of Orthopaedic Surgery, University of California Los Angeles, 1200 Rosecrans,
Suite 208, Manhattan Beach, CA 90266, USA*

The subtalar joint is a complex and functionally important joint of the lower extremity that plays a major role in the movement of inversion and eversion of the foot [1,2]. The complex anatomy of the subtalar joint makes arthroscopic and radiographic evaluation difficult. The development of arthroscopes with small diameters and excellent optical capacity along with precise techniques has allowed arthroscopy of the subtalar joint to expand. Anatomic portals and arthroscopic anatomy of the posterior subtalar joint in cadaveric specimens were first described by Parisien and Vangsness [3] in 1985. One year later, Parisien [4] published the first clinical report on subtalar arthroscopy, which evaluated three cases with good results. Since then, a number of reports on posterior subtalar arthroscopy and its clinical applications have become available. Lateral and posterior anatomic approaches have been used for performing posterior subtalar joint arthroscopy. Arthroscopic subtalar management has been credited with clear advantages for the patient, including faster postoperative recovery period, decreased postoperative pain, and fewer complications [5]. Although posterior subtalar arthroscopy is still met with some skepticism, the technique has slowly evolved as an alternative to open subtalar surgery.

No external funding and no benefits have been received by the authors. The authors report no competing interests.

* Corresponding author.
E-mail address: l.beimers@amc.uva.nl (L. Beimers).

Indications

Subtalar arthroscopy may be applied as a diagnostic and therapeutic instrument. The diagnostic indications for subtalar arthroscopy include persistent pain, swelling, stiffness, locking, or catching of the subtalar area resistant to all conservative treatment [5,6]. In addition, subtalar joint arthroscopy can be used for visual assessment of the subtalar articular surfaces when persistent pain is present after a chronic ankle sprain or a fracture of the os calcis [7]. Therapeutic indications for subtalar joint arthroscopy include debridement of chondromalacia, subtalar impingement lesions, excision of osteophytes, lysis of adhesions with post-traumatic arthrofibrosis, synovectomy, and the removal of loose bodies. Other therapeutic indications are instability, debridement and drilling of osteochondritis dissecans, retrograde drilling of cystic lesions, removal of a symptomatic os trigunum, and calcaneal fracture assessment and reduction [8,9]. Arthroscopic arthrodesis of the subtalar joint was introduced in 1994 [10].

Contraindications

Absolute contraindications to subtalar arthroscopy include localized infection leading to a potential septic joint and advanced degenerative joint disease, particularly with deformity. Relative contraindications include severe edema, poor skin quality, and poor vascular status.

Equipment and setup

Two different anatomic approaches are used for arthroscopy of the posterior subtalar joint. The arthroscope generally used for lateral subtalar joint arthroscopy is a 2.7-mm 30° short arthroscope (Box 1). Others prefer to use the 10° or 25° arthroscope of the same diameter for subtalar arthroscopy [8]. In addition, a 70° arthroscope can be helpful to look around corners and to facilitate instrumentation. In subtalar joints that are too tight to allow a 2.7-mm arthroscope, a 1.9-mm 30° arthroscope is advised. A small joint shaver set with a 2.0-and 2.9-mm shaver blade and small abrader is also needed.

For a two-portal posterior approach to the posterior subtalar joint, the instrumentation used is essentially the same as for knee joint arthroscopy (Box 2). With this technique, the subtalar joint capsule and the adjacent fatty tissue are partially resected. A sufficiently large working space adjacent to the joint is created, making it possible to use a 4.0-mm 30° arthroscope. The arthroscope is placed at the joint level and looks inside the joint without entering the joint space. The maximum size of the intra-articular instruments depends on the available joint space.

Box 1. Equipment for subtalar joint arthroscopy

1.9-mm, 2.7-mm 30° and 70° video arthroscopes, cannulae
2.0-mm, 2.9-mm full-radius blades, whiskers, and burrs
18-guage spinal needle
K-wires
Drill
Ring curettes, pituitary
Small joint probes and graspers
Normal saline and gravity system
Noninvasive distractor

Distraction of the subtalar joint can be accomplished with noninvasive and invasive methods. The type of distraction chosen depends on the tightness of the joint and the location of disease. Noninvase distraction during arthroscopy can be done manually by an assistant or by a noninvasive distraction strap around the hindfoot [11]. In most cases, joint distraction is obtained using normal saline and a gravity system. Regarding invasive joint distraction, using talocalcaneal distraction with pins inserted from laterally is a better choice than tibiocalcaneal distraction, especially with a tight posterior subtalar joint [12]. The disadvantage of using an invasive distractor is the potential damage to soft tissues (ie, the lateral calcaneal branch of the sural nerve) and ligamentous structures, the risk of fracturing the talar neck or body, and infection.

Subtalar joint anatomy

The subtalar joint can be divided, for arthroscopic purposes, into anterior (talocalcaneonavicular) and posterior (talocalcaneal) articulations (Fig. 1)

Box 2. Equipment for subtalar joint arthroscopy using the two-portal approach

4.0-mm 30° video arthroscope, cannulae
4.5-mm, 5.5-mm full-radius blades, whiskers, and burrs
21-guage needle
K-wires
Drill
Ring curettes, pituitary
Small joint probes and graspers
Normal saline and gravity system
Noninvasive distractor

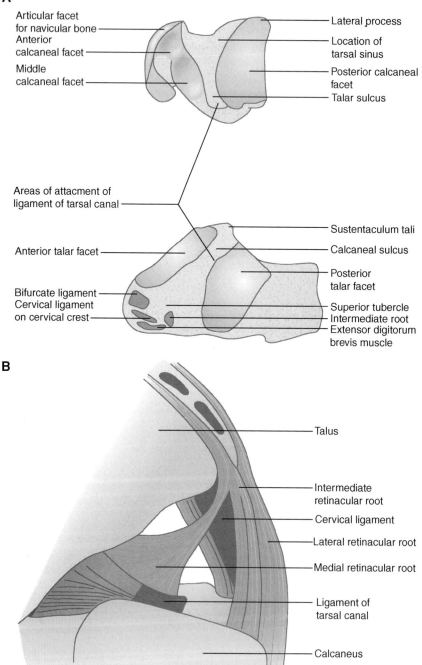

A

Articular facet
for navicular bone
Anterior
calcaneal facet
Middle
calcaneal facet

Lateral process
Location of
tarsal sinus
Posterior calcaneal
facet
Talar sulcus

Areas of attacment of
ligament of tarsal canal

Anterior talar facet

Bifurcate ligament
Cervical ligament
on cervical crest

Sustentaculum tali
Calcaneal sulcus
Posterior
talar facet
Superior tubercle
Intermediate root
Extensor digitorum
brevis muscle

B

Talus

Intermediate
retinacular root
Cervical ligament
Lateral retinacular root
Medial retinacular root
Ligament of
tarsal canal

Calcaneus

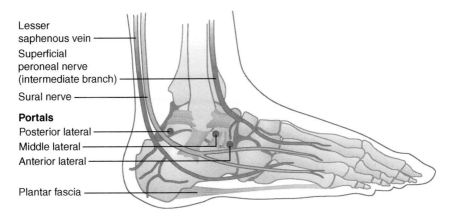

Lesser saphenous vein
Superficial peroneal nerve (intermediate branch)
Sural nerve
Portals
Posterior lateral
Middle lateral
Anterior lateral
Plantar fascia

Fig. 2. Anatomy of the lateral portal sites with the structures at risk.

[13–15]. The anterior and posterior articulations are separated by the tarsal canal; the lateral opening of this canal is called the sinus tarsi (a soft area ~2 cm anterior to the tip of the lateral malleolus). Within the tarsal canal, the medial root of the inferior extensor retinaculum, the cervical and talocalcaneal interosseous ligaments, fatty tissue, and blood vessels are found. The lateral ligamentous support of the subtalar joint consists of superficial, intermediate, and deep layers (Fig. 2) [6,16]. The superficial layer comprises the lateral talocalcaneal ligament, the posterior talocalcaneal ligament, the medial talocalcaneal ligament, the lateral root of the inferior extensor retinaculum, and the calcaneofibular ligament. The intermediate layer is formed by the intermediate root of the inferior extensor retinaculum and the cervical ligament. The deep layer comprises the medial root of the inferior extensor retinaculum and the interosseous ligament. The talocalcaneonavicular, or anterior subtalar joint, is composed of the talus, the posterior surface of the tarsal navicular, the anterior surface of the calcaneus, and the plantar calcaneonavicular, or spring ligament. The posterior talocalcaneal, or posterior subtalar joint, is a synovium-lined articulation formed by the posterior convex calcaneal facet of the talus and the posterior concave talar facet of the calcaneus. The joint capsule is reinforced laterally by the lateral talocalcaneal ligament and the calcaneofibular ligament. This joint also has a posterior capsular pouch with small lateral, medial, and anterior recesses. Arthroscopic visualization of the subtalar joint is limited to its posterior facet. The anterior portion of the subtalar joint is generally thought to be inaccessible to arthroscopic examination because of the thick ligaments that fill the sinus tarsi.

Fig. 1. (*A*) Anatomy of the subtalar joint. The talus is shown from under its surface and the calcaneus from above (superiorly). (*B*) Anatomy of the lateral subtalar joint with a view from posterior to anterior.

Portal placement and safety

Lateral approach

Access to the posterior subtalar joint can be achieved through a lateral approach and a posterior approach. Three portals are recommended for visualization and instrumentation of the subtalar joint using the lateral approach. The anatomic landmarks for lateral portal placement include the lateral malleolus, the sinus tarsi, and the Achilles tendon. The lateral malleolus is routinely palpable. The sinus tarsi is also usually palpable, although it can be filled with large amounts of adipose tissue [6]. Inversion and eversion of the foot may be helpful in palpating the sinus tarsi. The anterolateral portal is established approximately 1 cm distal to the fibular tip and 2 cm anterior to it (Figs. 3–5). Anatomic structures at risk with placement of the anterolateral portal include the dorsal intermediate cutaneous branch of the superficial peroneal nerve, the dorsal lateral cutaneous branch of the sural nerve, the peroneus tertius tendon, and a small branch of the lesser saphenous vein. The dorsal intermediate cutaneous branch of the superficial peroneal nerve is located an average of 17 mm anterior to the portal. The dorsolateral cutaneous branch of the sural nerve is located an average of 8 mm inferior to the portal [17]. The middle portal is described as being about 1 cm anterior to the tip of the fibula, directly over the sinus tarsi. The middle portal places no structures at risk during the course of its placement. The posterolateral portal is approximately 0.5 cm proximal to or at the fibular tip and just lateral to the Achilles tendon. Anatomic structures at risk with placement of the posterolateral portal for subtalar arthroscopy are the sural nerve, the small saphenous vein, and the peroneal tendons. In a study on portal safety, the posterior portal was located 4 mm posterior to the sural nerve in most cases [17]. Literature has also described accessory portals for posterior subtalar arthroscopy [6,18]. The accessory anterolateral and posterolateral portals are used as needed for viewing and instrumentation. The accessory anterolateral portal is usually slightly anterior and superior to the anterolateral portal. The accessory posterolateral portal is made behind the peroneal tendons, lateral to the posterolateral portal.

Posterior approach

Posterior subtalar arthroscopy can be performed using a posterolateral and posteromedial portal [19]. This two-portal endoscopic approach to the hindfoot with the patient in the prone position has been credited to offer better access to the medial and anterolateral aspects of the posterior subtalar joint [12,20]. The medial aspect of the posterior subtalar joint is tighter than on the lateral side, possibly increasing the risk of iatrogenic cartilage damage and necessitating the use of an invasive distractor [18]. The tibial nerve, the posterior tibial artery, and the medial calcaneal nerve can be at risk when the posteromedial portal is used [6,21]. Investigators studied the relative safety of the posterior portals for hindfoot endoscopy in anatomic specimens (Table 1) [12,21–23]. Mekhail and col-

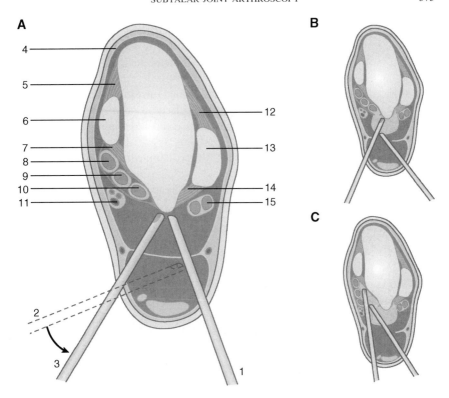

Fig. 3. (*A*) Cross-section of the ankle joint at the level of the arthroscope. 1, arthroscope placed through the posterolateral portal, pointing in the direction of the webspace between first and second toe; 2, full-radius resector introduced through the posteromedial portal until it touches the arthroscope shaft; 3, resector glides in an anterior direction until it touches bone; 4, crural fascia; 5, anterior superficial band of the deltoid ligament; 6, medial malleolus; 7, deep portion of the deltoid ligament; 8, posterior tibial tendon; 9, flexor digitorum tendon; 10, flexor hallucis longus tendon; 11, neurovascular bundle; 12, anterior talofibular ligament; 13, fibula; 14, posterior talofibular ligament; 15, peroneal tendons. (*B*) The arthroscope shaft is pulled backward until the shaver comes into view. The fatty tissue overlying the capsule of the talocrural joint and subtalar joint is removed. The flexor hallucis longus is used as a landmark; it is the medial border of the posterior working area. (*C*) The shaver and arthroscope are positioned in the area between the tarsal tunnel structures and the ankle joint. A posteromedial capsulectomy can be performed, and calcifications in this area or ossicles located posterior from the medial malleolus can be removed. The instruments can be brought into the posterior part of the ankle joint or subtalar joint when desired.

leagues [12] measured an average distance between the point of entry of the posteromedial arthroscope and the posterior tibial neurovascular bundle of 1.0 cm (the closest distance was 8 mm). Sitler and colleagues [22] evaluated the safety of posterior ankle arthroscopy with the use of posterior portals with the limb in the prone position in 13 cadaveric specimens. The average distance between the posteromedial cannula and the tibial nerve was 6.4 mm (range, 0–16.2 mm). In addition, the distance between the posterior tibial artery and the cannula averaged

9.6 mm (range, 2.4–20.1 mm) and the average distance between the cannula and the medial calcaneal nerve was 17.1 mm (range, 19–31 mm). The height of the posteromedial portal in relation to the tip of the lateral malleolus is an important determinant regarding the proximity of the relevant anatomic structures to the edge of the cannula. It is unfortunate that not all investigators specified this measure. Other factors that could explain the variety in outcome are the use of joint distraction and the size of the arthroscope. Compared with the conventional posterolateral portal, the posteromedial portal is essentially equidistant to the neurovascular structures. It appears that the posteromedial portal in hindfoot endoscopy is relatively safe and reproducible and can be used for the treatment of intra- and extra-articular hindfoot pathology. The main difference between the two techniques is that the 2.7-mm lateral approach for posterior subtalar arthros-

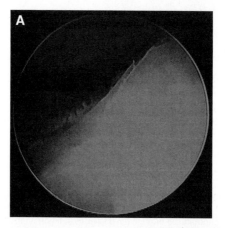

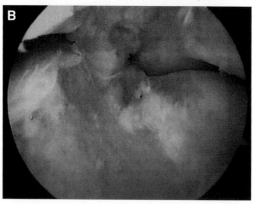

Fig. 4. Views of the subtalar joint as viewed from the anterior portal. (*A*) The anterior process of the calcaneus. (*B*) Posterior facet of subtalar joint (*left*) and anterior joint of subtalar (*right*) as seen through anterior portal. (Courtesy of Smith & Nephew, Andover, Massachusetts; with permission.) (*C*) The lateral capsule and lateral talocalcaneal ligament, arrow points to the lateral capsule. (*D*) Anterior joint of subtalar joint seen through anterior portal. (Courtesy of Smith & Nephew Dyonics, Andover, Massachusetts; with permission.)

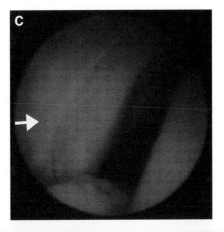

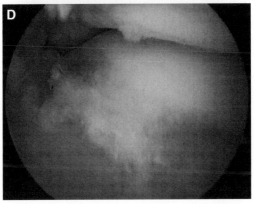

Fig. 4 (*continued*).

copy is a true arthroscopy technique in which the arthroscope and the instruments are placed within the joint, whereas the two-portal posterior technique (using a posterolateral and posteromedial portal) starts as an extra-articular approach. With the two-portal posterior technique, a working space is first created adjacent to the posterior subtalar joint by removing the fatty tissue overlying the joint capsule and the posterior part of the ankle joint. The joint capsule is then partially removed to be able to inspect the joint from outside-in, with the arthroscope positioned at the edge of the joint without entering the joint space. As mentioned earlier, the maximum size of the intra-articular instruments depends on the available joint space.

Surgical technique

Subtalar joint arthroscopy is performed with the patient under general or regional anesthesia. A tourniquet is applied to the proximal thigh and is inflated

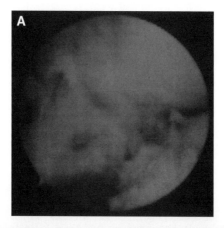

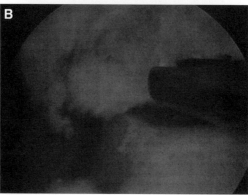

Fig. 5. (*A*) Sinus tarsi syndrome from interosseous ligament tear with impingement into the sinus tarsi and anterior aspect of the posterior joint. (*B*) Debridement of the interosseous ligament tear and impingement with a laser.

only when required for visualization. Using the lateral approach, the patient is placed in the lateral decubitis position with the operative extremity draped free. Padding is placed between the lower extremities and under the contralateral extremity to protect the peroneal nerve. The contralateral extremity is bent to 90° at the knee. The best portal combination for access to the posterior joint includes placement of the arthroscope through the anterior portal and the instrumentation through the posterior portal. This portal combination allows direct visualization and access of practically the entire surface of the posterior facet, the posterior aspect of the ligaments, the lateral capsule and its small recess, the os trigonum, and the posterior pouch of the posterior joint with its synovial lining. Instrumentation through the anterior portal provides access to the lateral aspect of the posterior facet. The medial, anterior, and posterior aspects cannot be reached well through the anterior portal. In addition, significant risk of iatrogenic damage to underlying subchondral bone exists. Access to the anterior and lateral portions of the posterior facet and structures located in the extra-articular sinus

Table 1
Posteromedial portal safety for posterior subtalar and hindfoot arthroscopy determined with anatomic dissection studies

Reference	No. of specimens	Achilles tendon	Flexor hallucis longus tendon	Tibial nerve	Posterior tibial artery	Medial calcaneal nerve
Feiwell and Frey, 1993 [21]	18	—	—	7.5 (0–13) [a]	12.6 (3–20) [a]	2.5 (0–6) [a]
Mekhail et al, 1995 [12]	6	—	—			
Sitler et al, 2002 [22]	13	0.6 (0–5.5)	2.7 (0–11.2)	6.4 (0–16.2)	9.6 (2.4–20.1)	17.1 (19–31)
Lijoi et al, 2003 [23]	10	—	—	13.3 (11–17)	17.3 (15–21)	14.7 (8–20)

Values are average distances (and range) to relevant anatomic structures measured in millimeters.

Abbreviation: —, not measured by authors.

[a] Tibial neurovascular bundle: 10 mm (at least 8 mm).

tarsi can also be obtained by placing the arthroscope through the anterior portal and instrumentation through the middle portal. In addition, excellent visualization of the medial and posterior aspects of the posterior facet is possible, even though they cannot be reached by instrumentation through the middle portal. This portal combination is recommended for visualization and instrumentation of the sinus tarsi and anterior aspects of the posterior subtalar joint.

The anterior portal is first identified with an 18-gauge spinal needle, and the joint is inflated with a 20-mL syringe. The needle is removed and a small skin incision made. The subcutaneous tissue is gently spread using a straight mosquito clamp. Using the same path, an interchangeable cannula with a semiblunt trocar is placed, followed by a 2.7-mm 30° oblique arthroscope. The middle portal is now placed under direct visualization using an 18-gauge spinal needle and outside-in technique. When visualized, the needle is removed and replaced with an interchangeable cannula. The posterior portal can be placed at this time using the same outside-in technique. It is easy to become disoriented while arthroscoping the posterior subtalar joint. The arthroscope may be placed inadvertently in the ankle joint or may penetrate the capsule of the ankle and enter the lateral ankle gutter. For this reason, fluoroscopic confirmation of the position of the arthroscope can be useful [24].

The technique of the two-portal endoscopic approach to the hindfoot using the posterolateral and posteromedial portals adjacent to the Achilles tendon should be performed as described here. The posterolateral portal is made at the level or slightly above the tip of the lateral malleolus, just lateral to the Achilles tendon. After making a vertical stab incision, the subcutaneous layer is gently split by a mosquito clamp. The mosquito clamp is directed anteriorly, pointing in the direction of the interdigital webspace between the first and second toe. When the tip of the clamp touches bone, it is exchanged for a 4.0-mm arthroscope shaft with blunt trocar pointing in the same direction. By palpating the bone in the sagittal plane, the level of the posterior subtalar joint can most often be distinguished by palpating the prominent posterior talar process. The posteromedial portal is made just medial to the Achilles tendon. In the horizontal plane, it is located at the same level as the posterolateral portal. After making the skin incision, a mosquito clamp is introduced and directed toward the arthroscope shaft. When the mosquito clamp touches the shaft of the arthroscope, the shaft is used as a guide to travel anteriorly in the direction of the posterior subtalar joint. All the way, the mosquito clamp must touch the arthroscope shaft until the mosquito clamp touches bone. The blunt trocar is exchanged for a 4.0-mm 30° arthroscope. The direction of view is to the lateral side to prevent damage to the lens system. The arthroscope is pulled slightly backward until the tip of the mosquito clamp comes into view. The clamp is used to spread the extra-articular soft tissue just in front of the tip of the arthroscope. The mosquito clamp can now be exchanged for a 4.5-mm full-radius resector to remove the subtalar joint capsule posterolaterally to visualize the joint. The next step is to remove the posterior talocalcaneal ligament to visualize the posterior and posteromedial part of the subtalar joint. In most cases, it is not possible to introduce the 4.0-mm arthroscope into the posterior subtalar joint; however, the posterior subtalar joint can be adequately visualized from its margins without entering the joint with the 4.0-mm arthroscope. At this time, intra-articular joint pathology can be treated under direct view looking from outside-in using small-sized instruments (Fig. 4).

After completing the arthroscopic procedure, the portals are closed with sutures. When there is extravasation of fluid into the subcutaneous tissue, the portals are sometimes left open so that the irrigation solution can escape. A compression dressing is applied from the toes to the midcalf. This dressing is removed the following day; ice is applied, with the leg elevated for 2 to 3 days. The patient is allowed to ambulate with the use of crutches, and weight bearing is permitted as tolerated. The sutures are removed approximately 1 week after the procedure, and the patient is encouraged to start range-of-motion exercises of the foot and ankle immediately after surgery. When the joint swelling has completely subsided, the patient, if indicated, is referred to a physical therapist for rehabilitation under supervision. The patient should be able to return to full activities at 6 to 12 weeks postoperatively.

Arthroscopic evaluation of the posterior subtalar joint

When performing diagnostic subtalar arthroscopy, it is imperative to have a reproducible and systematic method of anatomic review to consistently examine the entire joint. A standard 13-point arthroscopic evaluation of the posterior subtalar joint has been advocated by Ferkel [6] and Williams and Ferkel [25]. Diagnostic subtalar arthroscopy examination begins with the arthroscope viewing from the anterolateral portal. From the anterolateral portal, the interosseous talocalcaneal ligament is readily visualized. Medially, the deep interosseous ligament (evaluation area 1) is observed and, as the arthroscope is slowly withdrawn, the superficial interosseous ligament (evaluation area 2) is seen (Fig. 5). From the anterior portal, an assessment of the floor of the sinus tarsi may be made. When the arthroscopic lens is rotated more anteriorly, the anterior process of the calcaneus can be evaluated (Fig. 6). As the arthroscopic lens is rotated laterally, the anterior aspect of the posterior talocalcaneal articulation (evaluation area 3) is observed (see Fig. 6). Next, the anterolateral corner (evaluation area 4) is examined, and reflections of the lateral talocalcaneal ligament (evaluation area 5) (see Fig. 6) and the calcaneofibular ligament (evaluation area 6) are observed. The lateral talocalcaneal ligament is noted anterior to the calcaneofibular ligament. The arthroscopic lens may then be rotated medially, and the central articulation (evaluation area 7) is observed between the talus and the calcaneus. Finally, the posterolateral gutter (evaluation area 8) may be seen from the anterolateral portal. The arthroscope is then switched to the posterolateral portal and the inflow cannula is switched to the anterolateral portal. From this view, the interosseous ligament may be seen anteriorly in the joint. As the arthroscopic lens is rotated laterally, the lateral talocalcaneal ligament (evaluation area 5) and calcaneofibular ligament (evaluation area 6) reflections may again be observed and

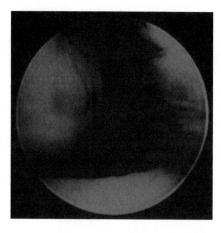

Fig. 6. Synovitis of the subtalar joint presenting as sinus tarsi syndrome.

their relationship noted. From this posterior view, the central talocalcaneal joint (evaluation area 7) may be examined and the posterolateral gutter (evaluation area 8) carefully assessed for synovitis and loose bodies. The posterolateral recess (evaluation area 9) and the posterior gutter (evaluation area 10) are then carefully evaluated in the normal bare area where the articulation ends and the posterior corner of the talus is assessed. The posteromedial recess (evaluation area 11) is carefully observed, and the posteromedial corner (evaluation area 12) of the talcocalcaneal joint and, finally, the most posterior aspect of the talcocalcaneal joint is seen (evaluation area 13). By rotating the arthroscope upward while keeping it in area 13, the os trigonum can be visualized on the talus (if present).

Results

Posterior subtalar arthroscopy has been shown to be beneficial over the past several years. Williams and Ferkel [25] collected information on 50 patients who had hindfoot pain who underwent simultaneous ankle and subtalar arthroscopy. Twenty-nine patients had subtalar pathology consisting of degenerative joint disease, subtalar dysfunction, chondromalacia, symptomatic os trigonum, arthrofibrosis, loose bodies, or osteochondritis of the talus that was treated arthroscopically. The anterolateral and posterolateral portals were used to visualize the posterior subtalar joint; distraction (invasive and noninvasive) was used in all cases. At an average follow-up of 32 months, these investigators reported good to excellent results in 86% of the patients. Overall, less favorable results were noted with associated ankle pathology, degenerative joint disease, age, and activity level of the patient. No operative complications were reported. Goldberger and Conti [26] retrospectively reviewed 12 patients who underwent subtalar arthroscopy for symptomatic subtalar pathology with nonspecific radiographic findings. The preoperative diagnoses were subtalar chondrosis in 9 patients and subtalar synovitis in 3 patients. The anterolateral and posterolateral portals were used to visualize the posterior subtalar joint. A femoral distractor was applied in patients when visualization was difficult. The follow-up averaged 17.5 months. The average preoperative American Orthopaedic Foot and Ankle Society (AOFAS) Hindfoot Score was 66 (range, 54–79); the average postoperative score was 71 (range, 51–85). In the 7 patients who improved after subtalar arthroscopy, the average improvement was 10 points on the AOFAS Hindfoot Score. Four patients' symptoms progressively worsened after surgery; all 4 were diagnosed as having grade 4 chondromalacia of the subtalar joint at the time of arthroscopy. Three of these patients progressed to subtalar arthrodesis at an average of 18 months following the arthroscopy. It is of interest that all patients stated that they would have the surgery again. In addition, 2 patients were very satisfied with the surgery, 6 patients were satisfied, and 4 patients were satisfied with reservations; none were dissatisfied. No operative complications occurred in this series. The investigators concluded that subtalar arthroscopy is the most accurate method of diagnosing subtalar articular cartilage damage but has limited therapeutic benefit in the treatment of early degenerative joint disease. The preoperative imaging studies tended to be less accurate predictors of subtalar cartilage damage than arthroscopy.

Sinus tarsi syndrome

Sinus tarsi syndrome was first described by O'Connor in 1958 [27]. It has historically been defined as persistent pain in the tarsal sinus secondary to trauma (80% of the cases reported) [28]. There are no specific objective findings in this condition. The exact etiology is not clearly defined, but scarring and degenerative changes to the soft-tissue structure of the sinus tarsi are thought to be the most common cause of pain in this region [6]. Walking on uneven terrain can result in pain and a feeling of instability. Clinical examination reveals pain on the lateral aspect of the hindfoot aggravated by firm pressure over the lateral opening of the sinus tarsi. Relief of symptoms with injection of local anesthetic directly into the sinus tarsi confirms the diagnosis. Surgical removal of the contents of the lateral half of the sinus tarsi improves or eradicates symptoms in roughly 90% of cases [29]. Kashuk and colleagues [18] stated that the application of arthroscopic techniques for decompression of the sinus tarsi has proved useful, is technically easy, and allows for a rapid recovery. Oloff and colleagues [28] presented 29 patients who underwent subtalar joint arthroscopy for sinus tarsi syndrome by way of an anterolateral approach. Subtalar joint synovectomy was the most common procedure performed; 12 patients had additional procedures. The mean postoperative AOFAS Hindfoot score was 85 (range, 59–100) and there were no complications. All 29 patients stated they were better after surgery and would undergo the procedure again without reservation. Earlier results and those of Oloff and colleagues [28] suggest that arthroscopic

A

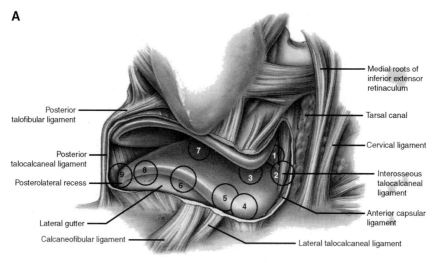

B

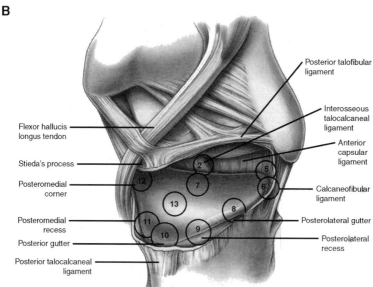

Fig. 7. (*A*) The 13-point arthroscopic evaluation of the posterior subtalar joint starts with a 6-point examination, viewed from the anterolateral portal. The posterior subtalar joint is examined starting at the most medial portion of the talocalcaneal joint, progressing laterally and then posteriorly. (*B*) Seven-point examination, viewed from the posterolateral portal. The posterior examination starts by visualizing along the lateral gutter, going posterolaterally, then posteriorly and medially, and ending centrally. (*Adapted from* Ferkel RD. Subtalar arthroscopy. Arthroscopic surgery: the foot and ankle. Philadelphia: Lippincott-Raven; 1996. with permission.)

synovectomy alone is associated with symptom resolution in patients who have sinus tarsi syndrome as opposed to the open methods that involve the removal of the entire lateral contents of the sinus tarsi. According to Frey and colleagues [30], sinus tarsi syndrome is an inaccurate term that should be replaced with a specific diagnosis because it can include many other pathologies such as interosseous ligament tears, arthrofibrosis (Fig. 7), synovitis, arthrofibrosis, and joint degeneration.

Os trigonum syndrome

The os trigonum is an unfused accessory bone found in close association with the posterolateral tubercle of the talus [31]. Impingement of the os trigonum, or os trigonum syndrome, is a common condition in ballet dancers and athletes and initiated by repetitive trauma. Symptomatology is caused by extreme plantar flexion, whereby the os trigonum is compressed between the posterior border of the tibia and the superior surface of the calcaneus. Clinically, pain can be elicited on palpation at the level of the posterior ankle joint and deep to the peroneal tendons. After failing appropriate nonoperative treatment, surgical excision of the bony impediment is recommended. Marumoto and Ferkel [32] performed a series of these arthroscopic procedures and reported favorable results in 11 patients after a mean follow-up period of 35 months. Ferkel [6] also reported successful use of the arthroscope in the management of symptomatic os trigonum. The excellent results of endoscopic removal of an os trigonum in 50 consecutive patients by means of the two-portal posterior hindfoot approach are presented by van Dijk in an article found elsewhere in this issue.

Arthroscopic subtalar arthrodesis

Arthroscopic subtalar arthrodesis was intended to yield less morbidity, preserve the blood supply, and preserve proprioception and neurosensory input [33]. The decision to proceed with this surgical technique grew out of the success with arthroscopic ankle arthrodesis. The main indications for arthroscopic subtalar arthrodesis include persistent and intractable subtalar pain secondary to degenerative osteoarthritis, rheumatoid arthritis, and post-traumatic arthritis [11,34–36]. Other indications include neuropathic conditions, gross instability, paralytic conditions secondary to poliomyelitis, and posterior tibial tendon rupture [37]. Factors that play a role in determining when arthroscopic subtalar arthrodesis is appropriate include the severity of the deformity and the amount of bone loss [11]. As with open subtalar arthrodesis, patients must have failed conservative treatment to qualify for arthroscopic subtalar fusion. The contraindications to this specific procedure are previously failed subtalar fusions, gross malalignment requiring correction, and significant bone loss [37].

In general, the procedure is performed as described here. The anterolateral and posterolateral portals are used in an alternating fashion during the procedure for viewing and for instrumentation. All debridement and decortication is performed posterior to the interosseous ligament. It is not as important to try to fuse the middle facet, although this can be done after resecting the contents of the sinus tarsi. The anterior facet of the subtalar joint is even more difficult to reach and is generally not fused. A primary synovectomy and debridement are necessary for visualization, as with other joints. Debridement and complete removal of the articular surface of the posterior facet of the subtalar joint down to subchondral bone is the next phase of the procedure. After the articular cartilage has been resected, approximately 1 to 2 mm of subchondral bone is removed to expose the highly vascular cancellous bone. Care must be taken not to remove excessive bone, which would lead to poor coaptation of the joint surfaces. After the subchondral plate is removed, small-spot-weld holes measuring approximately 2 mm in depth are created on the surfaces of the calcaneus and talus to create vascular channels. Careful assessment of the posteromedial corner must be made because residual bone and cartilage can be left there that can interfere with coaptation. The joint is then thoroughly irrigated of bone fragments and debris. In general, no autogenous bone graft or bone substitute is needed for this procedure. A joint defect and the sinus tarsi can be filled with small cancellous bone chips through an arthroscopic portal if desired. The foot is then put in the appropriate positions (about 0°–5° of hindfoot valgus) and the joint is compressed together. The fixation of the fusion is performed with a large cannulated self-drilling and self-tapping 6.5- or 7-mm lag screw. The guide pin is inserted from the dorsal anteromedial talus and angled posterior and inferior to the posterolateral calcaneus. It is important to place the guidewire under fluoroscopy with the ankle in maximum dorsiflexion to avoid any possible screw head impingement on the anterior lip of the tibia. Full weight bearing is allowed as tolerated at any time following surgery. In general, patients can tolerate full weight bearing without crutch support within 7 to 14 days after surgery. Tasto [37] advocated the use of a small lamina spreader through the anterolateral portal during the procedure to improve visualization and facilitate the maneuvering of surgical instruments. This technique has been successfully performed in patients who have primary degenerative joint disease of the subtalar joint without gross deformity or bone loss (Table 2).

Subtalar arthroscopy and treatment of calcaneal fractures

The development of wound complications is a major concern in the open reduction and internal fixation of displaced intra-articular calcaneal fractures [38]. Percutaneous, arthroscopically assisted screw osteosynthesis was developed to minimize the surgical approach without risking inadequate reduction of the subtalar joint. The method was applied in selected cases of displaced intra-articular

Table 2
Overview of arthroscopic subtalar arthrodesis

Reference	No. of patients	Main indications	Follow-up	Technique	Results[a]	Time until union	Complications
Jerosch, 1998 [41]	3	OA	3–5 mo	Supine, 4-portal, cancellous bone autograft	Excellent	3–5 mo	Algodystrophy (1)
Scranton, 1999 [34]	5	OA or PTA	4 had >1 y	Supine, 3-portal, talocalcaneal distraction	Excellent	6 mo	Screw removal (1)
Tasto, 2003 [37]	25	OA (8), PTA (10)	22 mo (6–92)	Lateral, 2-portal	Excellent	8.9 wk (6–16)	Screw removal (1)
Asou et al, 2003 [36]	6	PTA and ankle sprains	10 wk	Lateral, 2 cannulated screws	Excellent	10 wk	None

Postoperative regimens were different, possibly having an effect on the outcome.

Abbreviations: OA, osteoarthritis; PTA, post-traumatic arthritis.

[a] Parameters required for a successful arthrodesis were generally defined as evidence of bone consolidation across the subtalar joint, no motion or radiolucency at the screw tract, the clinical absence of pain with weight bearing, and pain-free forced inversion and eversion.

calcaneal fractures with one fracture line crossing the posterior calcaneal facet (Sanders type II fractures). Percutaneous leverage is performed with a Schanz screw introduced into the tuberosity fragment under direct arthroscopic and fluoroscopic control. The subtalar joint space is evaluated with respect to intra-articular displacement and position of the fragments by way of the posterolateral portal. When small chips or avulsion fragments are present, they can be removed through a second, anterolateral portal with a small grasper or shaver. After anatomic reduction is achieved, the fragments are fixed with three to six cancellous screws introduced by way of stab incisions. Gavlik and colleagues [39] treated 15 patients with this method and achieved good to excellent results in 10 patients, with a minimum of 1 year of follow-up.

Complications

The most likely complication to occur is an injury to any of the neurovascular structures in the proximity of the portals being used. Possible complications following subtalar joint arthroscopy include infection, instrument breakage, and damaging the articular cartilage. In addition, the use of invasive and noninvasive distraction devices can lead to various complications [40]. Because of the limited number of reports on posterior subtalar arthroscopy, no detailed information on the incidence of complications associated with this technique is available. In a series of 49 subtalar arthroscopic procedures using the lateral three-portal technique for treating various types of subtalar pathologic conditions, only five minor complications were reported [30]. There were three cases of neuritis involving branches of the superficial peroneal nerve. One patient had sinus tract formation and one had a superficial wound infection. Other studies report no complications with posterior subtalar arthroscopy; Ferkel evaluated 50 patients, with an average follow-up of 32 months (range, 16–51 months) and found no major complications following posterior subtalar arthroscopy. With arthroscopic arthrodesis of the subtalar joint, in two instances hardware problems were encountered requiring removal of the lag screw [34,37]. Jerosch [41] reported algodystrophy in one patient who was treated with arthroscopically assisted subtalar arthrodesis.

Summary

Diagnostic and therapeutic indications for posterior subtalar arthroscopy have increased. Subtalar arthroscopy can be performed using the lateral or the posterior two-portal technique, depending on the type and location of subtalar pathology. Arthroscopic subtalar surgery is technically difficult and should be performed only by arthroscopists experienced in advanced techniques. Arthroscopy of the subtalar joint and sinus tarsi is a valuable tool in the investigation of hindfoot pathology when conservative treatment fails and subtalar fusion is not indicated. There is a need for prospective clinical studies to provide data on the results and complications of subtalar arthroscopy.

References

[1] Inman VT. The subtalar joint. The joints of the ankle. Baltimore (MD): Williams & Wilkins Co.; 1976. p. 35–44.

[2] Perry J. Anatomy and biomechanics of the hindfoot. Clin Orthop 1983;177:9–15.

[3] Parisien JS, Vangsness T. Arthroscopy of the subtalar joint: an experimental approach. Arthroscopy 1985;1(1):53–7.

[4] Parisien JS. Arthroscopy of the posterior subtalar joint: a preliminary report. Foot Ankle 1986;6(5):219–24.

[5] Jaivin JS, Ferkel RD. Arthroscopy of the foot and ankle. Clin Sports Med 1994;13(4):761–83.

[6] Ferkel RD. Subtalar arthroscopy. Arthroscopic surgery: the foot and ankle. Philadelphia: Lippincott-Raven; 1996.

[7] Parisien JS. Arthroscopy of the posterior subtalar joint. In: Current techniques in arthroscopy. 3rd edition. New York: Thieme; 1998. p. 161–8.

[8] Parisien JS. Posterior subtalar joint arthroscopy. Guhl JF, Parisien JS, Boynton MD, editors. Foot and ankle arthroscopy. 3rd edition. New York: Springer-Verlag; 2004. p. 175–82.

[9] Cheng JC, Ferkel RD. The role of arthroscopy in ankle and subtalar degenerative joint disease. Clin Orthop Relat Res 1998;349:65–72.

[10] Lundeen RO. Arthroscopic fusion of the ankle and subtalar joint. Clin Podiatr Med Surg 1994;11(3):395–406.

[11] Stroud CC. Arthroscopic arthrodesis of the ankle, subtalar, and first metatarsophalangeal joint. Foot Ankle Clin 2002;7(1):135–46.

[12] Mekhail AO, Heck BE, Ebraheim NA, et al. Arthroscopy of the subtalar joint: establishing a medial portal. Foot Ankle Int 1995;16(7):427–32.

[13] Lapidus PW. Subtalar joint, its anatomy and mechanics. Bull Hosp Joint Dis 1955;16(2):179–95.

[14] Viladot A, Lorenzo JC, Salazar J, et al. The subtalar joint: embryology and morphology. Foot Ankle 1984;5(2):54–66.

[15] De Palma L, Santucci A, Ventura A, et al. Anatomy and embryology of the talocalcaneal joint. Foot Ankle Surg 2003;9:7–18.

[16] Harper MC. The lateral ligamentous support of the subtalar joint. Foot Ankle 1991;11(6):354–8.

[17] Frey C, Gasser S, Feder K. Arthroscopy of the subtalar joint. Foot Ankle Int 1994;15(8):424–8.

[18] Kashuk KB, Harmelin E, Holcombe R, et al. Arthroscopy of the ankle and subtalar joint. Clin Podiatr Med Surg 2000;17(1):55–79 [vi].

[19] Van Dijk CN, Scholten PE, Krips R. A 2-portal endoscopic approach for diagnosis and treatment of posterior ankle pathology. Arthroscopy 2000;16(8):871–6.

[20] Scholten PE, Altena MC, Krips R, et al. Treatment of a large intraosseous talar ganglion by means of hindfoot endoscopy. Arthroscopy 2003;19(1):96–100.

[21] Feiwell LA, Frey C. Anatomic study of arthroscopic portal sites of the ankle. Foot Ankle 1993; 14(3):142–7.

[22] Sitler DF, Amendola A, Bailey CS, et al. Posterior ankle arthroscopy: an anatomic study. J Bone Joint Surg Am 2002;84-A(5):763–9.

[23] Lijoi F, Lughi M, Baccarani G. Posterior arthroscopic approach to the ankle: an anatomic study. Arthroscopy 2003;19(1):62–7.

[24] Dreeben SM. Subtalar arthroscopy techniques. Oper Tech Sports Med 1999;7(1):41–4.

[25] Williams MM, Ferkel RD. Subtalar arthroscopy: indications, technique, and results. Arthroscopy 1998;14(4):373–81.

[26] Goldberger MI, Conti SF. Clinical outcome after subtalar arthroscopy. Foot Ankle Int 1998;19(7):462–5.

[27] O'Connor D. Sinus tarsi syndrome: a clinical entity. J Bone Joint Surg Am 1958;40:720–6.

[28] Oloff LM, Schulhofer SD, Bocko AP. Subtalar joint arthroscopy for sinus tarsi syndrome: a review of 29 cases. J Foot Ankle Surg 2001;40(3):152–7.

[29] Taillard W, Meyer JM, Garcia J, et al. The sinus tarsi syndrome. Int Orthop 1981;5(2):117–30.

[30] Frey C, Feder KS, DiGiovanni C. Arthroscopic evaluation of the subtalar joint: does sinus tarsi syndrome exist? Foot Ankle Int 1999;20(3):185–91.

[31] Chao W. Os trigonum. Foot Ankle Clin 2004;9(4):787–96 [vii].

[32] Marumoto JM, Ferkel RD. Arthroscopic excision of the os trigonum: a new technique with preliminary clinical results. Foot Ankle Int 1997;18(12):777–84.

[33] Tasto JP. Arthroscopic subtalar arthrodesis. In: Guhl JF, Parisien JS, Boynton MD, editors. Foot and ankle arthroscopy. 3rd edition. New York: Springer-Verlag; 2004. p. 183–90.

[34] Scranton Jr PE. Comparison of open isolated subtalar arthrodesis with autogenous bone graft versus outpatient arthroscopic subtalar arthrodesis using injectable bone morphogenic protein-enhanced graft. Foot Ankle Int 1999;20(3):162–5.

[35] Tasto JP, Frey C, Laimans P, et al. Arthroscopic ankle arthrodesis. Instr Course Lect 2000;49: 259–80.

[36] Asou E, Yamaguchi K, Kitahara H. Arthroscopic arthrodesis of subtalar joint: the new technique and short term results. Poster presented at the International Society of Arthroscopic Knee Surgery and Orthopaedic Sports Medicine Meeting. March 10–14, 2003.

[37] Tasto JP. Arthroscopic subtalar arthrodesis. Tech Foot Ankle Surg 2003;2(2):122–8.

[38] Gavlik JM, Rammelt S, Zwipp H. The use of subtalar arthroscopy in open reduction and internal fixation of intra-articular calcaneal fractures. Injury 2002;33(1):63–71.

[39] Gavlik JM, Rammelt S, Zwipp H. Percutaneous, arthroscopically-assisted osteosynthesis of calcaneus fractures. Arch Orthop Trauma Surg 2002;122(8):424–8.

[40] Ferkel RD, Small HN, Gittins JE. Complications in foot and ankle arthroscopy. Clin Orthop 2001;391:89–104.

[41] Jerosch J. Subtalar arthroscopy–indications and surgical technique. Knee Surg Sports Traumatol Arthrosc 1998;6(2):122–8.

ELSEVIER
SAUNDERS

Foot Ankle Clin N Am
11 (2006) 391–414

FOOT AND
ANKLE CLINICS

Hindfoot Endoscopy

C. Niek van Dijk, MD, PhD

Department of Orthopaedic Surgery, Academic Medical Center, P.O. Box 22660,
1100 DD Amsterdam, The Netherlands

Over the last 30 years, arthroscopy of the ankle joint has become an important diagnostic and therapeutic tool for chronic and post-traumatic ankle pain. Some investigators recommend routine placement of posterior portals in ankle arthroscopy [1–4]. In these cases, a posterolateral portal is recommended. A two-portal endoscopic approach to the hindfoot was first described in 2000 [5]. Hindfoot endoscopy gives excellent access to the posterior ankle compartment, the subtalar joint, and extra-articular structures such as the os trigonum, the deep portion of the deltoid ligament, the posterior syndesmotic ligaments, the tendons of the tarsal tunnel, the retrocalcaneal bursa, and the Achilles tendon [5]. This article describes indications and contraindications to hindfoot endoscopy, the operative technique, and the results of 146 endoscopic hindfoot procedures performed on 136 consecutive patients between 1994 and 2002 at the Academic Medical Center in Amsterdam, The Netherlands.

Indications and contraindications

Around the ankle joint, a variety of soft tissue pathologies can be present. In the absence of intra-articular damage, posteromedial ankle complaints are most often caused by disorders of the posterior tibial tendon [6]. In the event of failure of conservative treatment, posterior tibial tendon disorders can be treated by open surgery [7]. Posteromedial overuse and post-traumatic injuries in ballet dancers and soccer players most often are caused by tenosynovitis of the flexor hallucis longus tendon or a posterior impingement syndrome. Posterolateral ankle complaints most often are caused by disorders of the peroneal tendons, such as tenosynovitis, partial rupture, and tendon subluxation.

E-mail address: m.lammerts@amc.uva.nl

Articular pathology

Posterior compartment ankle joint

The main indications are the debridement and drilling of posteriorly located osteochondral defects of the ankle joint; removal of loose bodies, ossicles, post-traumatic calcifications or avulsion fragments; resection of posterior tibial rim osteophytes; treatment of chondromatosis; and treatment of chronic synovitis.

Posterior compartment subtalar joint

The main indications are osteophyte removal, removal of loose bodies, subtalar arthrodesis, and treatment of an intraosseous talar ganglion by drilling, curetting, and bone grafting.

Periarticular pathology

Posterior ankle impingement

Posterior ankle impingement is a pain syndrome. The patient experiences posterior ankle pain that is mainly present on forced plantar flexion. Posterior ankle impingement can be caused by overuse or trauma. Distinction between these two is important because posterior impingement through overuse has a better prognosis [8]. A posterior ankle impingement syndrome through overuse is mainly found in ballet dancers and runners [9–11]. Running that involves forced plantar flexion such as downhill running can put repetitive stress on the posterior aspect of the ankle joint [12]. In ballet dancers, the forceful plantar flexion during the *en pointe* position or the *demi-pointe* position cause compression at the posterior aspect of the ankle joint. The joint mobility and range of motion (ROM) gradually increases through exercise. In the presence of a prominent posterior talar process or an os trigonum, forceful plantor flexion can lead to compression of these structures (Fig. 1).

In 1995, the author and colleagues [9] reported on a group of 19 retired dancers after examining their ankle and subtalar joints. The mean length of the ballet dancers' professional careers was 37 years. All of the dancers had been dancing *en pointe*. None of these dancers had encountered a posterior ankle impingement syndrome. In 18 of the 38 investigated ankle joints, a hypertrophic posterior talar process or an os trigonum was present. The presence of an os trigonum itself does not seem to be relevant [9]. This anatomic anomaly must be combined with a traumatic event such as a supination trauma, a hyper–plantar flexion trauma, dancing on hard surfaces, or pushing beyond anatomic limits.

The forced hyper–plantar flexion test is most important for the diagnosis. With this test, the examiner performs a quick, passive, forced hyper–plantar flexion movement. The test can be repeated in slight exorotation or slight endorotation of the foot relative to the tibia. The investigator should apply this rotation movement on the point of maximal plantar flexion, thereby "grinding" the posterior talar process/os trigonum between the posterior tibial rim and calcaneus. The test is

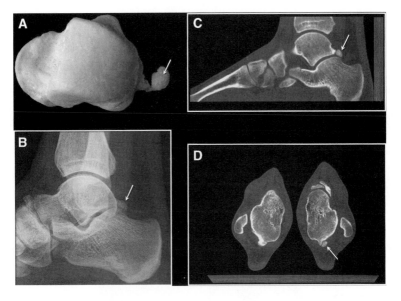

Fig. 1. Os trigonum (*arrows*). (*A*) Superior view of the right talus. (*B*) Lateral radiograph. (*C*) Sagittal CT scan. (*D*) Transverse CT scan.

positive when the patient has recognizable pain at the moment of impaction. A negative test rules out a posterior impingement syndrome. A positive test is followed by a diagnostic infiltration. If the pain on forced hyper–plantar flexion disappears, then the diagnosis is confirmed.

Deep portion of the deltoid ligament

Eversion or hyperdorsiflexion trauma can result in avulsion fragments, post-traumatic calcifications, or ossicles in the deep portion of the deltoid ligament (Fig. 2). Patients experience posteromedial ankle pain especially when running and walking on uneven ground.

Flexor hallucis longus

A flexor hallucis longus tendonitis is often present in patients who have a posterior ankle impingement syndrome. The pain is located posteromedially. In ballet dancers, it is present in plié and especially grand plié. The flexor hallucis longus tendon can be palpated behind the medial malleolus. By asking the patient to repetitively flex the big toe with the ankle in 10° to 20° of plantar flexion, the flexor hallucis longus tendon can be palpated in its gliding channel behind the medial malleolus. The tendon glides up and down under the palpating finger of the examiner. In cases of stenosing tendonitis or chronic inflammation, crepitus

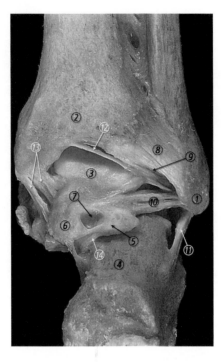

Fig. 2. Posterior view of the osteoarticular dissection of the ankle joint. 1, lateral malleolus; 2, tibia; 3, talus; 4, calcaneus; 5, lateral posterior talar process; 6, medial posterior talar process; 7, tendon sheath of flexor hallucis longus; 8, posterior tibiofibular ligament (superficial component); 9, transverse ligament or deep component of the posterior tibiofibular ligament; 10, posterior talofibular ligament; 11, calcaneofibular ligament; 12, posterior intermalleolar ligament or tibial slip; 13, superficial and deep layers of the collateral medial ligament of the ankle; 14; posterior talocalcaneal ligament.

and recognizable pain can be provoked. Sometimes a nodule in the tendon can be felt to move up and down under the palpating finger.

Neurovascular bundle

Entrapment of the posterior tibial nerve within the tarsal tunnel is commonly known as tarsal tunnel syndrome [13]. Clinical examination is sufficient to differentiate this disorder from an isolated posterior tibial tendon disorder.

Operative technique: posterior ankle arthroscopy (hindfoot endoscopy)

The procedure is performed as outpatient surgery under general anesthesia or epidural anesthesia. The patient is placed in a prone position. A tourniquet is applied around the upper leg and a small support is placed under the lower leg, making it possible to move the ankle freely. A soft tissue distraction device can be used when indicated [14].

For irrigation, normal saline is used, although glycine or Ringer's solution can also be used. One saline bag is used, with gravity flow. A 4.0-mm arthroscope with 30° is routinely used for posterior ankle arthroscopy. In addition to the standard excisional and motorized instruments for treatment of osteophytes and ossicles, a 4-mm chisel and periosteal elevator can be useful.

The landmarks on the ankle are the lateral malleolus, medial and lateral border of the Achilles tendon, and the foot sole. The ankle is kept in a neutral position. A straight line is drawn from the tip of the lateral malleolus to the Achilles tendon, parallel to the foot sole (Fig. 3).

The posterolateral portal is made just above this line, just in front of the Achilles tendon. After making a vertical stab incision, the subcutaneous layer is split by a mosquito clamp. The mosquito clamp is directed anteriorly, pointing in the direction of the interdigital webspace between the first and second toe. When the tip of the clamp touches the bone, it is exchanged for a 4.5-mm arthroscope shaft, with the blunt trocar pointing in the same direction. By palpating the bone

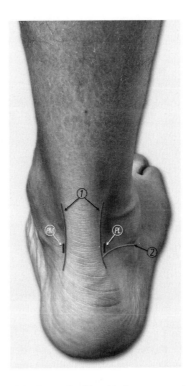

Fig. 3. Superoposterior view of the foot and ankle with the cutaneous landmarks for posterior ankle arthroscopy. 1, lateral and medial border of the Achilles tendon; 2, tip of lateral malleolus and a line drawn from the tip of the lateral malleolus to the lateral border of Achilles tendon, parallel to the foot sole. PL, Posterolateral portal; Posteromedial portal.

in the sagittal plane, the level of the ankle joint and subtalar joint can often be distinguished because the prominent posterior talar process or os trigonum can be felt as a posterior prominence between the two joints. The trocar is situated extra-articular at the level of the ankle joint. The trocar is exchanged for the 4-mm arthroscope; the direction of view is 30° to the lateral side.

The posteromedial portal is made at the same level, just above the line from the tip of the lateral malleolus, but just in front of the medial aspect of the Achilles tendon (see Fig. 3). After making a vertical stab incision, a mosquito clamp is introduced and directed toward the arthroscope shaft in a 90° angle. When the mosquito clamp touches the shaft of the arthroscope, the shaft is used as a guide to "travel" anteriorly in the direction of the ankle joint, all the way down, touching the arthroscope shaft until it reaches the bone. The arthroscope is now pulled slightly backward, sliding over the mosquito clamp until the tip of the mosquito clamp comes to view. The clamp is used to spread the extra-articular soft tissue in front of the tip of the lens (Fig. 4). In situations in which scar tissue or adhesions are present, the mosquito clamp is exchanged for a 5-mm full-radius shaver [5]. The tip of the shaver is directed in a lateral and slightly plantar direction toward the lateral aspect of the subtalar joint.

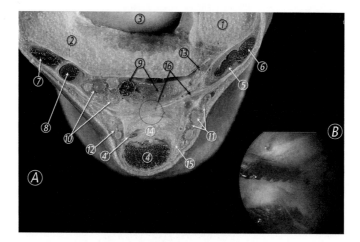

Fig. 4. (*A*) Macrophotography of the posterior area of the transverse section at the ankle joint level. 1, lateral malleolus; 2, tibia; 3, talus; 4, Achilles tendon; 4′, plantaris tendon; 5, peroneus brevis tendon; 6, peroneus longus tendon; 7, tibialis posterior tendon; 8, flexor digitorum longus tendon; 9, flexor hallucis longus tendon (musculotendinous); 10, tibial nerve and posterior tibial artery and veins; 11, sural nerve and short saphenous vein; 12, saphenous nerve and great saphenous vein; 13, anterior peroneal artery; 14, pre-Achilles tendon fat pad or Kager's triangle; 15, superficial crural fascia; 16, deep crural fascia or ligament of Rouvière and Canela. (*B*) Endoscopic image. The clamp is used to spread the extra-articular soft tissue in front of the tip of the lens at the level of pre-Achilles tendon fat pad.

The joint capsule and fatty tissue can be removed. After removal of the very thin joint capsule of the subtalar joint, the posterior compartment of the subtalar joint can be inspected. At the level of the ankle joint, the posterior tibiofibular ligament and the posterior talofibular ligament are recognized. The posterior talar process can be freed of scar tissue and the flexor hallucis longus tendon is identified (Fig. 5). The flexor hallucis longus tendon is an important landmark (Fig. 6). After removal of the thin joint capsule of the ankle joint, the ankle joint is entered and inspected.

On the medial side, the tip of the medial malleolus and the deep portion of the deltoid ligament are visualized. By opening the joint capsule from inside out at the level of the medial malleolus, the tendon sheath of the posterior tibial tendon can be opened and the arthroscope can be introduced into the tendon sheath. The posterior tibial tendon can be inspected. The same procedure can be followed for the flexor digitorum longus tendon.

By applying manual distraction to the os calcis, the posterior compartment of the ankle opens up and the shaver can be introduced into the posterior ankle

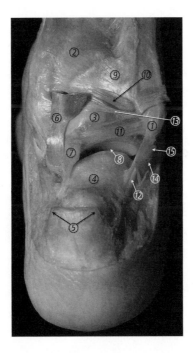

Fig. 5. Posterior view of the anatomic dissection of the ankle joint. 1, lateral malleolus (tip); 2, tibia; 3, talus; 4, calcaneus; 5, lateral and medial border of the Achilles tendon (cut); 6, flexor hallucis longus; 7, lateral posterior talar process; 8, posterior subtalar joint; 9, posterior tibiofibular ligament (superficial component); 10, transverse ligament or deep component of the posterior tibiofibular ligament; 11, posterior talofibular ligament; 12, calcaneofibular ligament; 13, posterior intermalleolar ligament or tibial slip; 14, peroneus longus tendon; 15, peroneus brevis tendon.

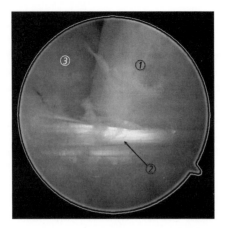

Fig. 6. Endoscopic view. 1, flexor hallucis longus tendon (important landmark); 2, fibrous component of the tendon sheath of flexor hallucis longus (flexor retinaculum); 3, lateral posterior talar process (os trigonum in case this is not attached to the talus).

compartment. The author prefers to apply a soft tissue distractor [14]. A total synovectomy or capsulectomy can be performed. The talar dome can be inspected over almost its entire surface, in addition to the complete tibial plafond. An osteochondral defect or subchondral cystic lesion can be identified, debrided, and drilled. The posterior syndesmotic ligaments are inspected and, when hypertrophic, partially resected.

Removal of a symptomatic os trigonum, a nonunion of a fracture of the posterior talar process, or a symptomatic large posterior talar prominence involves partial detachment of the posterior talofibular ligament and release of the flexor retinaculum, which both attach to the posterior talar prominence. Release of the

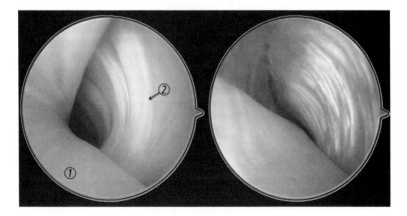

Fig. 7. Tendoscopy of the flexor hallucis longus tendon sheath. 1, flexor hallucis longus tendon; 2, fibrous component of the tendon sheath of flexor hallucis longus.

flexor hallucis longus tendon involves detachment of the flexor retinaculum from the posterior talar process. The tendon sheath can now be entered with the scope, following the tendon under the medial malleolus, and a further release can be performed (Fig. 7).

When a tight and thickened crural fascia is present, it can hinder the free movement of instruments. It can be helpful to enlarge the hole in the fascia by means of a punch or shaver. Bleeding is controlled by electrocautery at the end of the procedure.

After removal of the instruments, the stab incisions are closed with 3.0 non-absorbable suture to prevent sinus formation. A sterile compression dressing is applied.

Postoperative treatment consists of weight bearing, as tolerated, on crutches for 2 or 3 days. The dressing can be taken off after 3 days. As soon as possible after the surgery, the patient is advised to start ROM exercises, as tolerated.

Technical alternatives and pitfalls

In the hindfoot, the crural fascia can be thick. This local thickening is called the ligament of Rouvière (Fig. 8; see Fig. 4). It can be attached to the posterior talar process. It can be helpful to enlarge the entry through the crural fascia. The author uses an arthroscopic punch or scissors.

The position of the arthroscope is important. The operator should always check whether the direction of view is lateral. When the scope points into the direction of the webspace of the first and second toe, the scope is in a safe area. One should stay lateral of the flexor hallucis longus tendon and use the flexor hallucis longus tendon as a landmark. One should go medial from the flexor hallucis longus tendon only in cases in which a release of the neurovascular bundle is required (post-traumatic tarsal tunnel syndrome). When removing a

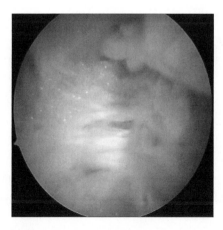

Fig. 8. Endoscopic view of the deep crural fascia or ligament of Rouvière and Canela.

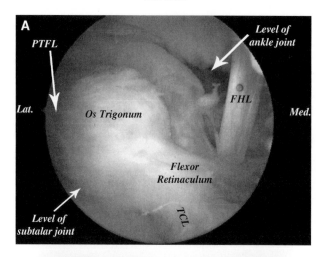

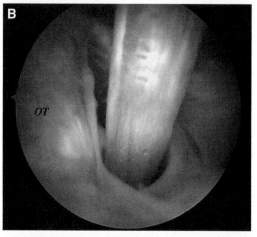

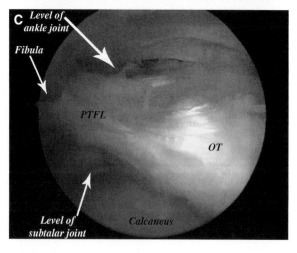

hypertrophic posterior talar process by chisel, the operator should take care not to place the chisel too far anterior but should start at the posterosuperior edge of the posterior talar process and chisel away the inferoposterior part of the process. The remnant of the process can be taken away by a shaver (bone cutter). If the chisel is placed too far anterior, then the subtalar joint can be entered.

The advantage of a two-portal procedure with the patient in the prone position is the working space between the Achilles tendon and the back of the ankle and subtalar joint. The position is ergonomic for the orthopedic surgeon. Soft tissue distraction can easily be applied [14].

An alternative is to use two posterolateral portals, with the patient in the lateral decubitus position [15]. The author has no experience with this approach.

Rehabilitation

The postoperative treatment consists of functional treatment. Most patients are advised to start practicing ROM immediately after surgery and protected weight bearing as tolerated for the first 3 days. One week postoperatively, patients are seen in the outpatient department. If necessary, physiotherapy can be prescribed for ROM, strengthening, and stability.

Patients

Between 1994 and 2002 at the Academic Medical Center in Amsterdam, 146 endoscopic hindfoot procedures were performed on 136 consecutive patients. The main indication was a posterior ankle impingement syndrome. In 52 patients, a bony impediment (os trigonum or hypertrophic posterior talar process) was removed. In 28 patients, a posterior ankle impingement syndrome was combined with a flexor hallucis longus tendinitis (Figs. 9, 10). Apart from removal of the bony impediment, release of the flexor hallucis longus was performed (Table 1). In 8 patients, the cause of the posterior ankle impingement syndrome was a soft tissue impediment, which was removed by a shaver. In total, 44 patients had a flexor hallucis longus tendinitis. There was an isolated flexor hallucis longus tendonitis in only 7 patients, whereas in the other patients, the

---

Fig. 9. Endoscopic view of the posterior aspect of the left ankle in a patient who had a symptomatic os trigonum and flexor hallucis longus tendonitis. (A) Os trigonum with its connection to the posterior talofibular ligament (PTFL), the flexor retinaculum, and the talocalcaneal ligament (TCL). FHL, flexor hallucis longus; Lat., lateral; Med., medial. (B) Focusing at the medial aspect of the os trigonum (OT) showing its connection with the flexor retinaculum. (C) Focusing at the lateral aspect of the OT showing its connection to the PTFL.

flexor hallucis longus tendinitis was combined with a bony impingement syndrome (28 patients) or an avulsion fracture of the posteromedial tibial rim (Fig. 11) or an ossicle near the flexor hallucis longus tendon (4 patients). The flexor hallucis longus tendinitis was combined with posteromedial talar osteochondral defect in 5 patients.

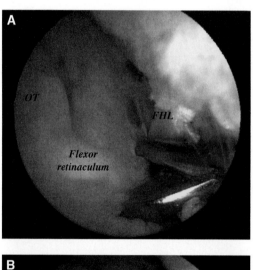

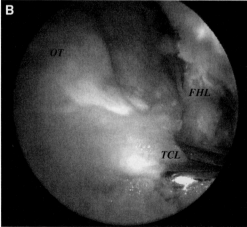

Fig. 10. Endoscopic procedure for removing an os trigonum (OT) and releasing the flexor hallucis longus (FHL) in a left ankle. (*A*) Cutting through the flexor retinaculum. TCL, talocalcaneal ligament. (*B*) Cutting through the TCL. (*C*) Releasing the PTFL. (*D*) Overview of the OT released from its related anatomic structures. (*E*) Lifting of the OT with a probe. (*F*) Releasing the OT from its connection to talus by means of a small periosteal elevator (rasparatorium). (*G*) Removing the released OT. (*H*) Postoperative overview. IML, intermalleolar ligament.

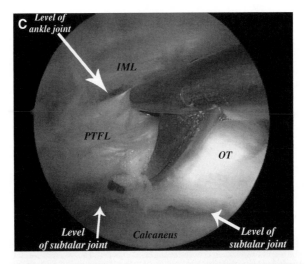

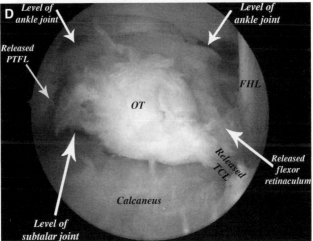

Fig. 10 (*continued*).

Hindfoot endoscopy for treatment of posterior ankle joint pathology was performed in 36 patients (Table 2). In 13 patients, an osteochondral defect was debrided and drilled. In 7 patients, the osteochondral defect was located at the posteromedial talar dome; in 4 patients, it was located in the tibial plafond; and in 2 patients, it was in the posterolateral talar dome. Post-traumatic calcifications in

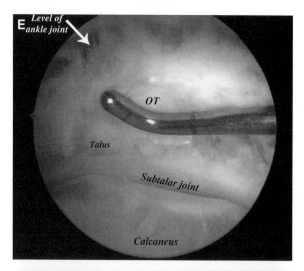

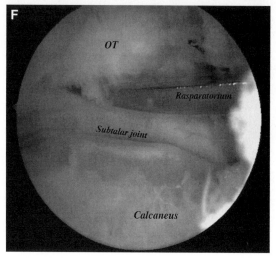

Fig. 10 (*continued*).

the posteromedial capsule or the posteromedial deltoid ligament were present in 5 patients. Two patients had a Cedell fracture (avulsion flexor retinaculum). All calcifications were removed endoscopically. In 9 patients, a total synovectomy was performed. The posterior synovectomy was performed first. The knee was flexed and an anterior synovectomy was performed by means of the standard

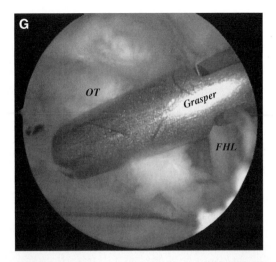

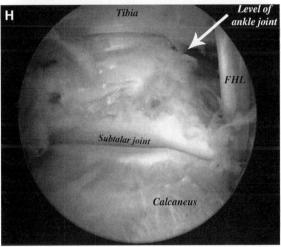

Fig. 10 (*continued*).

anterolateral and anteromedial approach. The indication was chondromatosis (2 patients), pigmented villunodular synovitis (3 patients), rheumatoid arthritis (2 patients), and cristal synovitis (2 patients).

A two-portal hindfoot endoscopy for subtalar pathology was performed for degenerative articular changes (10 patients) or removal of a loose body (1 patient),

Table 1
Endoscopy for periarticular hindfoot pathology: indications and procedures

No. of patients	Diagnosis	Treatment
8	Soft tissue impingement	Resection of soft tissue impediment
24	BI	Resection of os trigonum
28	BI + FHL tendinitis	Resection of OT + release FHL
7	FHL tendinitis	Release of FHL
4	FHL tendinitis + ossicle	Release of FHL + ossicle removal
5	FHL tendinitis + OD	Release of FHL + OD drilling
2	Tarsal tunnel syndrome	Release of tarsal tunnel

Abbreviations: BI, bony impingement; FHL, flexor hallucis longus; OD, osteochondral defect; OT, os trigonum.

whereas in 3 patients, a large talar intraosseous ganglion was treated. These multicystic lesions originated from the subtalar joint. By means of the two-portal hindfoot approach, the chondral defect (origin of the ganglion) in the subtalar joint was identified. The ganglion then was drilled through the posterior talar process. The drill hole was enlarged to 4.5 mm to make introduction of a currette possible. After curretting and drilling, the cystic defect was filled with cancellous bone from the iliac crest. Another procedure that can be performed by means of this two-portal hindfoot approach is subtalar arthrodesis (Fig. 12).

Results

There were no complications other than 2 patients who experienced a small area of diminished sensation over the heelpad of the hindfoot. Removal of a pathologic os trigonum or a painful posterior soft tissue impediment did not cause any technical problems and was successful in most patients (see Table 1). In

Table 2
Hindfoot endoscopy for posterior ankle/subtalar joint pathology: indications and procedures

No. of patients	Diagnosis	Treatment
13	Osteochondral defect ankle joint	Debridement + drilling
5	Loose body ankle joint	Removal of loose body
7	Calcification/avulsion	Removal of ossicles
2	Osteophyte posterior tibial rim	Resection of osteophytes
2	Chondromatosis	Anterior + posterior removal
7	Chronic synovitis	Anterior + posterior synovectomy
10	Degenerative changes subtalar joint	Osteophyte removal + debridement
1	Loose body subtalar joint	Removal
3	Intraosseus talar ganglion	Drilling, curetting, + grafting

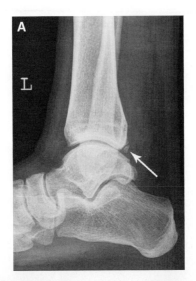

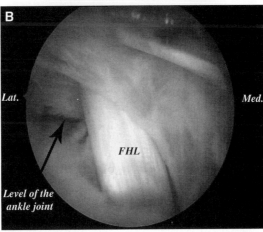

Fig. 11. Endoscopic procedure for removing an ununited posterior distal tibial rim fragment after a fracture. Patient presented with posterior left ankle pain. (*A*) Lateral (L) radiograph showing the ununited posterior distal tibial rim fragment (*arrow*). (*B*) Locating the flexor hallucis longus (FHL) and the level of the ankle joint. Lat., lateral; Med., medial. (*C*) Opening of the posterior ankle joint capsule and displacing the capsule and FHL medially with a hook. The ununited posterior distal rim fragment can now be identified. (*D*) Removing the fragment by way of the posteromedial portal. (*E*) Postoperative view showing the former location of the fragment and damage to the posterior superomedial talar surface that was caused by impingement of the slightly displaced fragment.

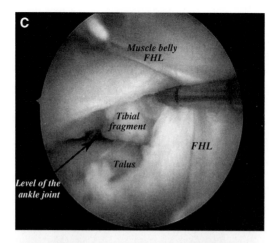

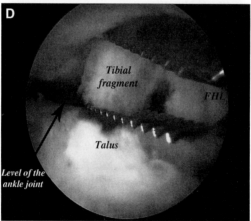

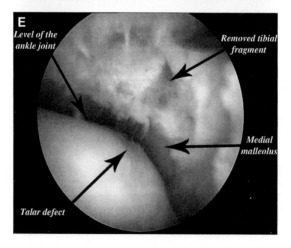

Fig. 11 (*continued*).

patients in whom a total synovectomy was performed, there was no recurrence of the synovitis. All loose bodies were successfully removed. Nine of the 13 debrided/drilled osteochondral defects had a good or excellent result. The 3 patients who had treatment of an intraosseous talar ganglion were without symptoms at the last follow-up. All patients who were treated for degenerative changes in the

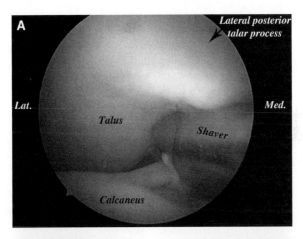

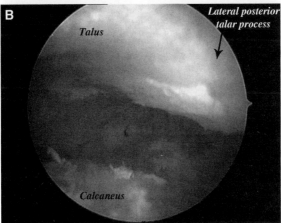

Fig. 12. Arthroscopic subtalar arthrodesis in a patient who had subtalar arthrosis in the left ankle. (*A*) Introducing the 5.5-mm shaver to create intra-articular workspace and to remove the cartilage. Lat., lateral; Med., medial. (*B*) Intra-articular view showing the bare calcaneal and talar surfaces (by means of a shaver and curette). (*C*) Damaging the subchondral plate with multiple grooves using a chisel. (*D*) Final situation before placing the screws. (*E*) Introduction of the first guidewire inside the subtalar joint under direct vision. (*F*) Postoperative radiograph.

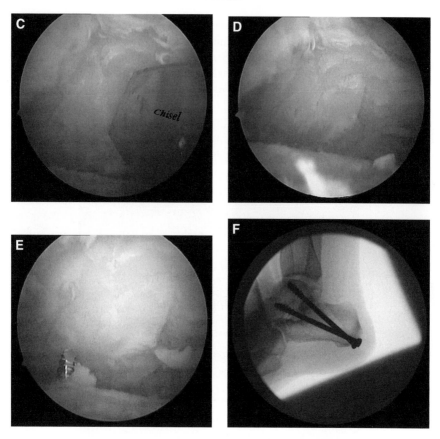

Fig. 12 (*continued*).

subtalar joint experienced a clear improvement of their symptoms. None of these patients had deterioration of the result over time (see Table 2).

Discussion

Posterior ankle impingement is a common cause of posterior ankle pain. It is a clinical diagnosis whereby the patient experiences pain in the hindfoot when the ankle is forced into a plantar-flexed position. The cause can be a trauma or overuse. Trauma can be hyper–plantar flexion or a combined inversion plantar flexion injury. The overuse injuries occur typically in ballet dancers and downhill runners. On physical examination, these patients have pain on palpation on the posterolateral aspect of the talus. The forced hyper–plantar flexion test is positive. After failure of conservative treatment, the impediment (os trigonum, scar tissue, hypertrofic posterior talar process, or ossicle) can be removed by means of an open posterolateral or posteromedial procedure [8,10,11,16–23]. The studies of Hamilton and colleagues [10] and Marotta and Micheli [19] dealt mainly with ballet dancers. Hamilton and colleagues [10] reported a good or excellent result in 30 of 40 (75%) open operations for posterior impingement syndrome and flexor hallucis longus tendonitis, with 15% complications. Marotta and Micheli [19] studied 12 patients, with 17% complications. In their patients, full-performance dancing was realizable at a mean of 3 months, with sporadic pain in 67% of cases. In dancers, overuse is presumably the cause in most cases. Sport resumption has been reported to take place after 13 to 25 weeks [10,19]. Abramowitz and colleagues [23] described the result of operative treatment in 41 patients who had posterior impingement. Overall, full recovery time averaged 5 months. Complications occurred in 10 of 41 patients (24%), and the average postoperative American Foot and Ankle Society (AOFAS) score was 87.6. The author's results compare favorably with these results. In the combined post-traumatic and overuse group, the author found an average recovery time for sports activities of 9 weeks and an AOFAS score of 90 at follow-up. The author found a 1% complications rate that corresponded to a small area of hypoerthesia in the heelpad. This complication rate compares favorably with the 9% complications rate reported by Ferkel and colleagues [24] occurring in foot and ankle arthroscopy in general, and with the rate of 15% to 24% found in the literature for open surgery in posterior ankle impingement [10,19,21,23].

   The use of an anterolateral portal combined with a posterolateral or subtalar portal is an alternative to approach the posterior compartment of the ankle joint. When combined with anterior ankle arthroscopy, most surgeons regard the posteromedial portal to be contraindicated in all but the most extreme situations because of the potential of serious complications. The posterolateral portal, however, is advocated as a routine portal by most investigators. The two-portal posterior endoscopic ankle approach with the patient in prone position offers excellent access to the posterior compartment of the ankle joint, the posterior subtalar joint, the flexor hallucis longus, and the os trigonum. When the arthroscope shaft is in place through the posterolateral, the introduction of instruments through the posteromedial portal must be directed toward the arthroscope shaft. The arthroscope shaft is then used as a guide for the medial instruments to travel in the direction of the joint. The neurovascular bundle is thus passed without problem. When performed in this manner, posterior ankle arthroscopy is a safe, reliable, and exciting method to diagnose and treat a variety of posterior ankle problems. It is recommended that the procedure be performed by an experienced arthroscopist who has studied the local anatomy in a cadaver setting. Reports on arthroscopic resection of a symptomatic os trigonum are few [25,26]. Marumoto and Ferkel [25] used an anterolateral and posterolateral portal in a study of 11 patients, with good results.

As was stated earlier by Stibbe and colleagues [8], in the open approach for posterior ankle impingement, overuse patients do better than patients who have impingement after a traumatic event. The author also found a larger improvement in AOFAS hindfoot score, better patient satisfaction, and less reduction in Tegnerscore in the overuse group compared with the post-traumatic group in endoscopically treated patients. Furthermore, return to work and sports activities was quicker in patients treated for overuse than for post-traumatic causes. The better outcome in patients who have an overuse syndrome can be partly explained by the additional injuries to the ankle structures in patients who have a post-traumatic impingement syndrome. This additional pathology is most likely the reason for residual complaints in these patients [8]. Patients who are treated for a bony impingement do better than patients who are treated for a soft tissue impingement. Misdiagnosis in soft tissue impingement is more likely to occur than in bony impingement. Furthermore, recurrence of scar tissue postoperatively is another potential reason for failure. Because of the close relation of the flexor hallucis longus tendon to the posterior talar process/os trigonum, tendinitis of the flexor hallucis longus is often present in patients who have a posterior impingement of the ankle. In the author's group, 63% had symptomatic involvement of the tendon. In a bony impingement, the flexor hallucis longus tendon can become irritated by a slight displacement of the os trigonum, by reactive synovitis, by capsular hypertrophy, or by scar tissue in this area. This association had no influence on prognosis. Sural nerve injury is the main complication in open posterolateral surgery for posterior ankle impingement [20,23]. In the author's group, two cases with a small area of hypoesthesia of the postermedial heelpad were found. Innervation to the medial retromalleolar region is variable [27]. No permanent loss of nerve function or neuroma formation was seen.

Summary

Treatment of posterior ankle impingement by means of a two-portal endoscopic hindfoot approach compares favorably to open surgery. Hindfoot endoscopy causes less morbidity and facilitates a quick recovery. When performed in the manner described in this article, posterior ankle arthroscopy is a safe, reliable, and exciting method to diagnose and treat a variety of posterior ankle problems. It is recommended that the procedure be performed by an experienced arthroscopist who has studied the local anatomy in a cadaver setting.

Acknowledgments

The author thanks Pau Golanó, MD, of the Laboratory of Arthroscopic and Surgical Anatomy, Department of Pathology and Experimental Therapeutics (Human

Anatomy Unit), University of Barcelona, Barcelona, Spain, and P.A.J. de Leeuw, PhD fellow, for recording and editing the arthroscopic/endoscopic images.

References

[1] Ferkel RD, Scranton PE. Current concepts review: arthroscopy of the ankle and foot. J Bone Joint Surg Am 1993;75:1233–42.

[2] Guhl JF. Foot and ankle arthroscopy. New York: Slack; 1993.

[3] Andrews JR, Timmerman LA. Diagnostic and operative arthroscopy. Philadelphia: WB Saunders; 1997.

[4] Ferkel RD. Arthroscopic surgery. In: Whipple TL, editor. The foot and ankle. New York: Lippincott-Raven; 1996.

[5] Van Dijk CN, Scholten PE, Krips R. A 2-portal endoscopic approach for diagnosis and treatment of posterior ankle pathology. Arthroscopy 2000;16(8):871–6.

[6] Myerson M. Tendons and ligaments in current therapy. In: Myerson M, editor. Current therapy in foot and ankle surgery. St. Louis: Mosby-Year Book; 1993. p. 123–35.

[7] Lapidus PW, Seidenstein H. Chronic non-specific tenosynovitis with a fusion about the ankle. J Bone Joint Surg 1950:175–9.

[8] Stibbe AB, Van Dijk CN, Marti RK. The os trigonum syndrome. Acta Orthop Scand 1994; (Suppl 262):59–60.

[9] Van Dijk CN, Lim LSL, Poortman A, et al. Degenerative joint disease in female ballet dancers. Am J Sports Med 1995;23(3):295–300.

[10] Hamilton WG, Geppert MJ, Thompson FM. Pain in the posterior aspect of the ankle in dancers. J Bone Joint Surg Am 1996;87:1491–500.

[11] Hedrick MR, McBryde AM. Posterior ankle impingement. Foot Ankle Int 1994;15:2–8.

[12] Funk DA, Cass JR, Johnson KA. Acquired adult flatfoot secondary to posterior tibial tendon pathology". J Bone Joint Surg Am 1986;68(1):95–102.

[13] Coughlin MJ, Mann RA. Tarsal tunnel syndrome. In: Surgery of the foot and ankle, vol. 1. 6th edition. St. Louis (MO): Mosby; 1993.

[14] Van Dijk CN, Verhagen RA, Tol HJ. Technical note: resterilizable noninvasive ankle distraction device. Arthroscopy 2001;17(3):E12:1–5

[15] Lundeen RO. Arthroscopic excision of the os trigonum. In: Guhl JF, Parisien JS, Boyton MD, editors. Foot and ankle arthroscopy. 3rd edition. New York: Springer-Verlag; 2004. p. 191–9.

[16] Van Dijk CN, Stibbe AB, Marti RK. Posterior ankle impingement. In: Nyska M, Mann G, editors. The unstable ankle. Human Kinetics. New York: Springer-Verlag; 2002. p. 139–48.

[17] Wenig JA. Os trigonum syndrome. J Bone Joint Surg Am 1990;80(5):278–82.

[18] Bruns J, Eggers-Stroder G. Das Os-Trigonum-Syndrom [The os trigonum syndrome]. Sportverletz Sportschaden 1991;5(3):155–8.

[19] Marotta JJ, Micheli LJ. Os trigonum impingement in dancers. Am J Sports Med 1992;20:533–6.

[20] Veazy BL, Heckman JD, Galindo MJ, et al. Excision of ununited fractures of the posterior process of the talus: a treatment for chronic posterior ankle pain. Foot Ankle 1992;13(8):453–7.

[21] Callanan I, Williams L, Stephens M. "Os post peronei" and the posterolateral nutcracker impingement syndrome. Foot Ankle Int 1998;19(7):475–8.

[22] Zeichen J, Schratt E, Bosch U, et al. Das Os-Trigonum-Syndrom [the os trigonum syndrome]. Unfallchirurg 1999;102:320–3.

[23] Abramowitz Y, Wollstein R, Barzilay Y, et al. Outcome of resection of a symptomatic os trigonum. J Bone Joint Surg Am 2003;85:1051–7.

[24] Ferkel RD, Small HN, Gittins JE. Complications in foot and ankle arthroscopy. Clin Orthop Rel Res 2001;391:89–104.

[25] Marumoto JM, Ferkel RD. Arthroscopic excision of the os trigonum: a new technique with preliminary clinical results. Foot Ankle Int 1997;18(12):777–84.

[26] Lombardi CM, Silhanek AD, Connolly FG. Modified arthroscopic excision of the symptomatic os trigonum and release of the flexor hallucis longus tendon: operative technique and case study. J Foot Ankle Surg 1999;38(5):347–51.

[27] Aszmann OC, Ebmer JM, Dellon AL. Cutaneous innervation of the medial ankle: an anatomic study of the saphenous, sural and tibial nerves and their clinical significance. Foot Ankle Int 1998;19(11):753–6.

ELSEVIER
SAUNDERS

Foot Ankle Clin N Am
11 (2006) 415–420

FOOT AND
ANKLE CLINICS

Tendoscopy of the Peroneal Tendons

Peter E. Scholten, MD[a],*, C. Niek van Dijk, MD, PhD[b]

[a]Kliniek Klein Rosendael, Department of Orthopaedic Surgery, Rosendaalselaan 30,
6891 DG Rozendaal, The Netherlands
[b]Department of Orthopaedic Surgery, Academic Medical Center, P.O. Box 22660,
1100 DD Amsterdam, The Netherlands

Post-traumatic lateral ankle pain is seen frequently. Peroneal tendon pathology is not always recognized as a cause of lateral ankle pain. Peroneal tendon disorders are often associated with and secondary to chronic lateral ankle instability. Because the peroneal muscles act as lateral ankle stabilizers, more strain is placed on these tendons in chronic lateral ankle instability, resulting in hypertrophic tendinopathy, in tenosynovitis, and ultimately in (partial) tendon tears [1–3]. Diagnosis may be difficult in a patient who has lateral ankle pain. Peroneal tendon dislocation and tenosynovitis can be established by clinical examination. Supplemental investigations such as MRI and sonography may be helpful in confirming the diagnosis [1] in cases of (subtotal) tears of the peroneus brevis or longus tendons. Postsurgery and post-traumatic adhesions and irregularities in the posterior aspect of the fibula (ie, tendon sliding channel) can also be responsible for symptoms in this region.

Pathology consists of tenosynovitis of the peroneal tendons, tendon dislocation or subluxation, and (partial) rupture or snapping of one or both of the peroneal tendons, and accounts for most symptoms at the posterolateral side of the ankle joint [4,5]. Rheumatoid tenosynovitis or a bony spur can also be the cause of posterolateral ankle pain. A differentiation must be made with (fatigue) fractures of the fibula, lesions of the lateral ligament complex, and posterior impingement of the ankle (os trigonum syndrome).

The primary indication for treating peroneal tendon disorders is pain. Nonsurgical treatment is usually attempted first. Conservative therapy includes activity modification, footwear changes, temporary immobilization, and corticosteroid injection. Lateral heel wedges can take stress off of the peroneal tendons to allow

---

* Corresponding author.
E-mail address: pscholten@medinova.com (P.E. Scholten).

1083-7515/06/$ – see front matter © 2006 Elsevier Inc. All rights reserved.
doi:10.1016/j.fcl.2006.03.004

healing. Failure of conservative measures is an indication for operative intervention. In contrast to arthroscopy, which has become the major technique to
treat intra-articular ankle lesions, extra-articular pathology of the ankle has traditionally demanded open surgery. This type of intervention frequently requires
postoperative plaster immobilization to prevent equinus malformation and to
stimulate wound healing [3,6]. Open ankle surgery may be complicated by injury
to the sural nerve or superficial peroneal nerve, infection, scarring, and stiffness
of the ankle joint [7–9]. The occurrence of these complications stimulated the
development of extra-articular endoscopic techniques. These techniques potentially lack the previously described disadvantages. Extra-articular ankle endoscopy has been developed in the last years, especially hindfoot endoscopy and
tendoscopy of the posterior tibial and peroneal tendons [10–12]. Endoscopic
ankle surgery is followed by a functional postoperative treatment and offers the
advantages of less morbidity, reduction of postoperative pain, and outpatient
surgery [12].

An anatomic study was performed to study the local anatomy of the peroneal
tendons and its surroundings and to verify portal anatomy [10,11]. In seven
cadaver ankles, the relation of the peroneal tendons to each other, to the posterolateral aspect of the distal fibula, and to the lateral aspects of the calcaneus
and cuboid was studied. The peroneus brevis tendon is situated dorsomedial of
the peroneus longus tendon from its proximal aspect up to the fibular tip with
a flattened constitution. Just distally to this lateral malleolus tip, the peroneus
brevis tendon gets a round aspect and crosses the round peroneus longus tendon.
The posterolateral part of the fibula forms a sliding channel for the two peroneal
tendons. This malleolar groove is formed by a periosteal cushion of fibrocartilage
that covers the bony groove. The tendons are held in their position within the
malleolar groove by the superior peroneal retinaculum. In three of the seven
lateral ankle explorations, a bony prominence on the calcaneus was found in
between both tendons some 4 to 5 cm distal from the fibula. A 1- to 2-mm thick

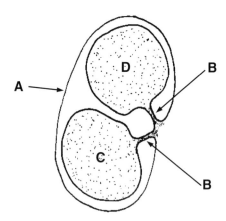

Fig. 1. Schematic drawing of a cross-section of the peroneal tendons with their tendon sheath and
vincula. A, tendon sheath; B, vincula; C, peroneus longus tendon; D, peroneus brevis tendon.

vinculum-like membrane was found between the peroneus longus and brevis tendons, dorsally attached to the dorsolateral aspect of the fibula (Fig. 1). The distal fibers of the peroneus brevis muscle belly gradually transform to this membraneous layer to end approximately at the tip of the fibula. At the peroneus longus site of this membrane, it is continuously attached to the peroneus brevis tendon, from its distal muscle fibers (6 to 9 cm proximally from the fibular tip), around the tip, and all the way to its distal insertion. It was found that access to the tendon sheath can be made all along the curse of the tendons proximally some 6 cm from the posterior tip of the lateral malleolus and distally about 3 cm from the fibular tip.

This article describes the technique and results of peroneal tendoscopy performed in 23 patients between 1995 and 2000.

Surgical technique

The patient is placed in supine position. The operation is performed as an outpatient procedure under general, regional, or local anesthesia. Local anesthesia has the advantage of a possible dynamic investigation. Before the anesthesia is administered, the patient is asked to actively evert his or her foot. The tendon can be palpated, and the location of the portals are drawn onto the skin. When local anesthesia is used, the anesthetic is administered around the portals and into the tendon sheath. A support is placed under the ipsilateral buttock, and a tourniquet is inflated. Access to the tendons can be obtained anywhere along the tendons. A distal portal is made first, 2.0 to 2.5 cm distal to the posterior edge of the lateral malleolus. An incision is made through the skin covering the tendons. The tendon sheath is penetrated with an arthroscopic shaft with blunt trocar, and a 2.7-mm 30° inclination angle arthroscope is introduced (Fig. 2). A spinal needle is placed 2.0 to 2.5 cm proximal to the posterior edge of the malleolus under direct vision, creating a proximal portal directly over the tendons. Instruments like a probe, a disposable cutting knife, scissors, or a shaver system can be introduced. Through the distal portal, a complete overview can be obtained of both peroneal tendons. The inspection starts some 6 cm proximal from the posterior tip of the lateral malleolus where a thin membrane splits the tendon compartment into two separate tendon chambers. More distally, both tendons lie in one compartment. By rotating the endoscope over and in between both tendons, the complete compartment can be inspected. When a total synovectomy of the tendon sheath is to be performed, it is advisable to create a third portal more distal or more proximal than the portals described previously. In cases of recurrent dislocation of the peroneal tendons, fibular groove deepening can be performed endoscopically. Inspection typically reveals a partial detachment of the superior peroneal retinaculum and some scarring and tenosynovitis of the peroneal tendons at the level of the tip of the distal fibula. Using a probe, the tendons can be dislocated to inspect the distal retromalleolar groove. A small burr (3.2 mm) is introduced distally with the arthroscope proximally, and the retromalleolar groove is deep-

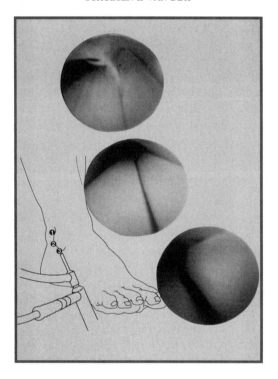

Fig. 2. Peroneal tendoscopy of the left ankle: the two main portals are located 2.0 to 2.5 cm proximal and 2.0 to 2.5 cm distal to the posterior edge of the lateral malleolus. 1, proximal portal; 2, lateral malleolus; 3, distal portal.

ened approximately 3 mm in depth and 5 mm in width. By relocating the tendons into the groove, the operator can check whether sufficient bone has been removed. At the end of the procedure, the tendons cannot be dislocated out of the groove. Because the superior peroneal retinaculum is partially stripped off the fibula and not torn, it can be expected to heal at its anatomic site without requiring further reattachment or postoperative plaster cast immobilization.

Both portals are sutured to prevent sinus formation, and a bandage is placed. Full weight bearing is allowed as tolerated. Active range of motion is advised immediately post surgery.

Results

Between 1995 and 2000, a peroneal tendoscopy was performed in 23 patients, with a minimum of 2 years' follow-up (Table 1). Eleven patients had a longitudinal rupture of the peroneal brevis tendon. In these patients, there was a history of an acute lateral ankle ligament rupture. Eight of these patients presented with pain and swelling over the posterior aspect of the lateral malleolus;

Table 1
Diagnosis and treatment of 23 patients in whom peroneal tendoscopy was performed between 1995 and 2000

No. of patients	Indication	Procedure
11	Longitudinal rupture of the peroneal brevis tendon	Tendoscopic synovectomy and suturing (miniopen)
10	Chronic tenosynovitis after operative treatment	Tendoscopic synovectomy (one removal of an exostosis)
2	Recurrent peroneal tendon dislocation	Tendoscopic fibular groove deepening

three presented a snapping sensation at the level of the lateral malleolus. Ten patients had persisting symptoms after operative treatment of a lateral malleolar fracture, a lateral ankle ligament reconstruction, or a surgical repair for recurrent tendon dislocation. Surgery consisted of an endoscopic tenosynovectomy, adhesiolysis, removal of an exostosis, and suturing a longitudinal rupture when indicated by way of a miniopen procedure.

Two patients had a tendoscopic deepening of the fibular groove for recurrent peroneal tendon dislocation. In one patient, the malleolar groove was concave; in the other patient, it was flat. The superior retinaculum was stripped off with the periosteum from the fibula (Fig. 3) and was not torn. This finding is in concordance with the earlier findings of peroneal tendon dislocation by Eckert and Davis [13]. After deepening the malleolar groove, peroneal tendon dislocation could no longer occur, allowing the superior retinaculum and fibular periosteum to attach at its original anatomic site and not require any further reattachment. Both patients did not require a plaster cast and after treatment were functional.

In these patients, the authors found no complications and no recurrence of the preoperative pathology.

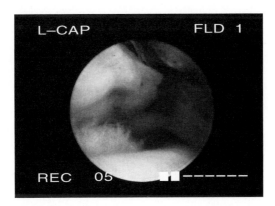

Fig. 3. Endoscopic view of the superior retinaculum and fibula on the left and the peroneal tendons on the right.

Summary

Tendoscopy of the peroneal tendons is a useful tool to diagnose and treat peroneal tendon disorders. Synovectomy, adhesiolysis, or removal of an exostosis can be performed endoscopically with low morbidity and an excellent functional outcome. Fibular groove deepening for recurrent tendon dislocation was successful in the two patients in whom this procedure was performed.

References

[1] Yao L, Tong JF, Cracchiolo A, et al. MR findings in peroneal tendopathy. J Comput Assist Tomogr 1995;19:460–4.

[2] Myerson M. Tendons and ligaments. In: Decker BC, editor. Current therapy in foot and ankle surgery. St. Louis: Mosby-Yearbook Inc.; 1993. p. 87–123.

[3] Richardson EG. Disorders of tendons. In: Grenshaw AH, editor. Campbell's operative orthopaedics. St. Louis (MO): CV Mosby Co.; 1992. p. 2851–73.

[4] Roggatz J, Urban A. The calcareous peritendinitis of the long peroneal tendon. Arch Orthop Trauma Surg 1980;96:161–4.

[5] Schweitzer GJ. Stenosing peroneal tenovaginitis. Case reports. S Afr Med J 1982;4:521–3.

[6] Lapidus PW. A note on the fracture of the os trigonum. Bull Hosp Joint Dis 1972;33:150–4.

[7] Marotta JJ, Micheli LJ. Os trigonum impingement in dancers. Am J Sports Med 1992;20:533–6.

[8] Hamilton WG, Geppert MJ, Thompson FM. Pain in the posterior aspect of the ankle in dancers. J Bone Joint Surg Am 1996;78:1491–500.

[9] Abramowitz Y, Wollstein R, Barzilay Y, et al. Outcome of resection of a symptomatic os trigonum. J Bone Joint Surg Am 2003;85:1051–7.

[10] van Dijk CN, Scholten PE, Kort NP. Tendoscopy (tendon sheath endoscopy) for overuse tendon injuries. Oper Techn Sports Med 1997;5:170–8.

[11] van Dijk CN, Kort NP. Tendoscopy of the peroneal tendons. Arthroscopy 1998;14(5):471–8.

[12] van Dijk CN. Hindfoot endoscopy. Sports Med Arthrosc Rev 2000;8:365–71.

[13] Eckert WR, Davis Jr EA. Acute rupture of the peroneal retinaculum. J Bone Joint Surg Am 1976;58(5):670–2.

ELSEVIER
SAUNDERS

Foot Ankle Clin N Am
11 (2006) 421–427

FOOT AND
ANKLE CLINICS

Tendoscopy of the Posterior Tibial Tendon

Gythe H. Bulstra, MD[a],[*], Paul G.M. Olsthoorn, MD[b],
C. Niek van Dijk, MD, PhD[a]

[a]*Department of Orthopaedic Surgery, Academic Medical Center, University of Amsterdam,
PO Box 22660, 1100 DD Amsterdam, The Netherlands*
[b]*Slotervaart Hospital, PO Box 90440, 1006 BK Amsterdam, The Netherlands*

Ankle joint disorders can be intra-articular or extra-articular. In the absence of intra-articular pathology, posteromedial ankle complaints are most often caused by a disorder of the posterior tibial tendon. The posterior tibial tendon can be subject to a number of pathologic conditions. Two predominant groups with a dysfunction of the tendon can be distinguished: the first group involves younger patients who may present with some form of systemic inflammatory disease; the second group involves older patients whose dysfunction is caused by chronic overuse [1]. Although the exact etiology of the disorder is unknown, the condition has been classified on the basis of clinical and radiographic findings. In the early stages of dysfunction, patients describe discomfort medially along the course of the tendon in addition to fatigue and aching on the plantar medial aspect of the ankle. In the presence of tenosynovitis, swelling is common. By clinical examination, a valgus angulation of the hindfoot and abduction of the forefoot can be seen and a "too-many-toes" sign is described [2]. For radiographs, MRI scanning is the best method for assessing a ruptured tendon. Investigation by means of ultrasound is recognized as a cost-effective and accurate method for evaluating disorders of the tendon [3].

Inactivity of the posterior tibial tendon gives midtarsal instability. The relative strength of the posterior tibial tendon is more than twice that of the peroneus brevis, its primary antagonist. Without the activity of the posterior tibial tendon, there is no stability at the midtarsal joint, and the forward propulsive force of the complex of gastrocsoleus acts at the midfoot instead of at the metatarsal heads. A total dysfunction eventually leads to a flatfoot deformity.

---

* Corresponding author.
E-mail address: bulstra@planet.nl (G.H. Bulstra).

1083-7515/06/$ – see front matter © 2006 Elsevier Inc. All rights reserved.
doi:10.1016/j.fcl.2006.03.001

Pain complaints are often located in the relative hypovascular zone immediately distal to the medial malleolus at 14 mm. The hypovascular zone may contribute to the development of degenerative changes and consequent ruptures. Van Dijk and colleagues [4] described the vincula that connect the posterior tibial tendon with its tendon sheath. Damage to the vincula can cause thickening, shortening, and scarring of the distal free edge. In post-traumatic, postsurgery, and postfracture situations, the vincula can be thickened and become symptomatic. In these patients, a painful local thickening can be palpated posterior and just proximal of the tip of the medial malleolus. Most dysfunctions of the tendon eventually lead to a painful tenosynovitis. The treatment is conservative in the beginning, including rest combined with immobilization using plaster or tape and nonsteroidal anti-inflammatory drugs. There is no consensus whether to use steroid injections; ruptures have been described. If conservative treatment fails, then operative treatment can be indicated. An open synovectomy is performed by means of sharp dissection, completely removing all the inflamed synovium while preserving the blood supply of the tendon. Postoperative management includes plaster cast immobilization for 3 weeks followed by wearing a boot with controlled ankle movement for another 3 weeks and physiotherapy [5]. Tenosynovitis is a common extra-articular manifestation of rheumatoid arthritis. Systemic inflammatory disease in the hindfoot in rheumatoid arthritis is a significant cause of disability for patients. Tenosynovitis in rheumatoid patients eventually leads to a ruptured tendon. In a group of patients who had rheumatoid arthritis and hindfoot pathology, Michelson and colleagues [6] found a dysfunction of the posterior tibial tendon in 13% to 64% depending on the specific diagnostic criteria. The criteria used were loss of the longitudinal arch, inability to perform a heel-rise, or lack of a palpable posterior tibial tendon. It is well known that arthroscopic synovectomy is preferred when arthroscopic access allows radical synovectomy [7]. Previous successful endoscopical synovectomy has been described [4,8,9]. An endoscopic procedure offers the advantage of less morbidity, reduction of the postoperative pain, and outpatient treatment [4,10]. This article illustrates endoscopy of the posterior tibial tendon in a diverse group of patients.

Surgical technique

The patient is placed in supine position. A tourniquet is placed on the affected leg. Before the anesthesia is administered, the patient is asked to actively invert the foot. The posterior tibial tendon can be palpated and the two portals are marked onto the skin. The operation can be performed under general, regional, or local anesthesia. Access to the tendon can be obtained anywhere along the course of the tendon; however, the two main portals are located directly over the tendon 2.0 cm distal and 2.0 to 4.0 cm proximal to the posterior edge of the medial malleolus (Fig. 1). The distal portal is made first: the incision is made through the skin only, and the tendon sheath is penetrated by the arthroscopy shaft with a blunt trocar. The 2.7-mm arthroscope with an inclination angle of 30° is

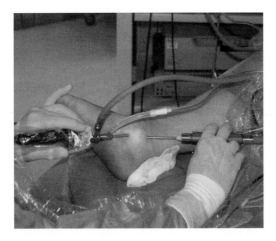

Fig. 1. Position of the scope during the operation.

introduced, and the tendon sheath is filled with saline. Under direct visualization, the proximal portal is made by introduction of a spinal needle and, subsequently, an incision is made through the skin into the tendon sheath. Instruments such as blunt probes, scissors, retrograde knife, and shaver system can be introduced (Fig. 2). For a rheumatoid arthritis synovectomy, a 3.5-mm shaver can be used. Synovectomy can be performed under the complete overview of the tendon from the distal portal over the insertion of the navicular bone to some 6 cm above the tip of the medial malleolus. The complete tendon sheath can be inspected by rotating the scope around the tendon. Special attention is given to inspect the tendon sheath covering the deltoid ligament, the posterior medial malleolus surface, and the posterior ankle joint capsule. At the end of the procedure, the portals are sutured. Postoperative treatment consists of a pressure bandage and

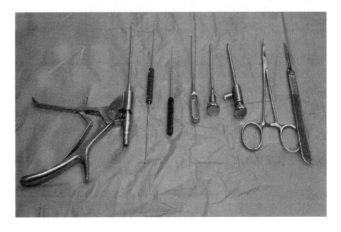

Fig. 2. Instruments used for the operative procedure.

partial weight bearing for 2 to 3 days. Active movements are stimulated from the first day. The operation is performed as an outpatient procedure. The procedure can easily be combined with other operations like arthroscopic synovectomy of the ankle or corrective surgery of the forefoot.

Patients

Between 1994 and 1997, the authors performed 16 procedures on 16 patients (7 women, 9 men). The average age was 33.6 years (range, 16–54 years). The right ankle was involved in 9 cases. All patients had a history of persistent posteromedial ankle pain for at least 6 months, with pain on palpation of the posterior tibial tendon, positive resistance test results, and often local swelling. The indications were diagnostic procedure after surgery in 5 patients, diagnostic procedure after fracture in 5, diagnostic procedure after trauma in 1, chronic tenosynovitis in 2, screw removal medial malleolus in 1, and posterior ankle arthrotomy in 2 patients (Fig. 3).

Between 1997 and 2004, the authors performed 19 procedures in 17 patients (11 women, 6 men). The average age was 43 years (range, 22–73 years). Ten endoscopic synovectomy procedures were performed in 8 patients who had chronic tenosynovitis due to rheumatoid arthritis (6 women, 2 men). All had a history of persistent posteromedial ankle pain, with pain on palpation of the posterior tibial tendon, positive resistance test results, and local swelling. All patients were initially treated with conservative therapy such as immobilization (plaster and orthopedic shoes) and noninflammatory drugs, and some had steroid injections in the tendon sheath. All patients had temporary pain relief. The patients were treated by the rheumatologist for their rheumatoid arthritis with systemic therapy.

In all eight patients, the diagnosis of synovitis without a rupture of the tendon was confirmed by means of ultrasound or MRI. In three patients, the endoscopy

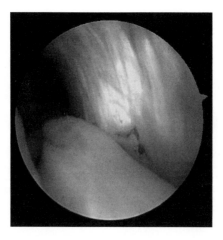

Fig. 3. A superficial tear of the posterior tibial tendon.

Table 1
Diagnosis and treatment of 33 patients in whom an endoscopic procedure of the posterior tibial tendon was performed between 1994 and 2004

No. of patients	Diagnosis	Treatment
10	Tenosynovitis due to rheumatoid arthritis	Tenosynovectomy
1	Healed medial malleolus fracture	Screw removal
1	Exostosis sliding channel	Exostosis removal
21	No specific diagnosis	Various[a]

[a] In this diagnostic group, 4 patients had a pathologic, thickened vinculum that was resected, 6 patients had a longitudinal rupture that was sutured using a minimal open approach, 4 patients had degenerative tendon changes that were debrided, 3 had adhesions that were removed, and 3 patients had a synovitis that required a synovectomy.

was combined with an arthroscopical synovectomy of the ankle (two patients) or a hallux valgus correction. All patients were allowed full weight bearing without support after the operation, except for the patient who had the hallux valgus correction. All patients were able to exercise the ankle function postoperatively.

In the other nine patients, tendoscopy of the posterior tibial tendon was performed for miscellaneous reasons (Table 1).

Results

The average follow-up of the patients who were operated between 1994 and 1997 was 1.1 years (range, 4 months to 2 years). No complications were observed. In two patients, the tendon sheath of the flexor digitorum longus was entered first, without consequences. Three patients showed a pathologic, thickened vinculum, which was removed. Four patients showed adhesions, which were also removed. Two patients showed irregularity of the sliding channel, which was smoothed out (Fig. 4).

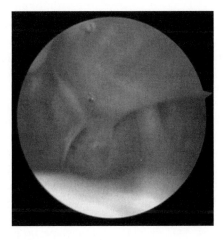

Fig. 4. The endoscopic view of a normal vinculum.

At follow-up, three of the four patients who had resection of pathologic vincula and two patients who underwent tenosynovectomy and tendon release were free of symptoms. Of the three patients whose adhesions were removed, one had a good result with diminished pain but the other two were not relieved of their symptoms. Of the seven patients in whom adhesions or a pathologic vinculum was removed, five subjectively experienced improvement in dorsiflexion of the ankle; however, in none could an increase of more than 5° be measured.

In the group of eight patients who underwent an endoscopical tenosynovectomy to treat chronic tenosynovitis in rheumatoid arthritis, the minimal follow-up was 1 year (range, 1–5 years). No complications where observed. In seven patients, an abundant synovitis was seen and removed. All patients had an intact tendon, with only superficial damage.

At follow-up of the eight patients, four had no recurrence of the synovitis and were fully satisfied with the outcome of the procedure. All had an intact tendon function and were able to stand tiptoe on one foot.

Two patients had a recurrence (at 9 months and at 18 months), both without a rupture of the posterior tibial tendon. Both patients successfully received a second endoscopic procedure after which they became symptom-free. Neither of these patients showed a too-many-toes sign at later follow-up.

Two patients were eventually less satisfied; one underwent a hindfoot arthrodesis after 2.5 years due to the arthritis of the hindfoot. One patient had remaining pain after the procedure without the development of a flatfoot deformity.

In the group of patients who were operated for miscellaneous reasons, there were no complications. All patients were satisfied about the operation itself. They were especially satisfied with the lack of postoperative pain, the early mobilization, the nice wound healing, and the quick recovery.

Discussion

The posterior tibial tendon plays an important role in normal hindfoot function. Post-traumatic and postsurgical complaints of pain at the posterior margin of the medial malleolus often pose a difficult diagnostic and therapeutic problem. In absence of intra-articular pathology, adhesions and irregularity in the tendon sliding channel can be responsible for symptoms in this region.

Post-traumatic posterior tibial dysfunction can lead to peritendinitis. Tenosynovitis can be (1) the result of overuse, (2) age related in seronegative spondylarthropathies, or (3) a part of rheumatoid arthritis. Open tendon release often requires postoperative plaster immobilization with the consequent possibility of new adhesion formation [5,11]. Endoscopic synovectomy of the posterior tibial tendon is not a difficult procedure when anatomic landmarks and proper portals are identified. Use of an endoscope allows direct visual assessment of the tendon and its sheath. In comparison with the open approach, this technique probably causes fewer adhesions. This diagnostic and therapeutic procedure can be performed as an outpatient procedure under local anesthesia and allows function after treatment and quick recovery. In addition, the risk of neurovascular damage is small.

Tendoscopy of the posterior tibial tendon proved to be successful in tendon sheath release, synovectomy, and removal of pathologic thickened vincula. The authors recommend endoscopy of the posterior tibial tendon for patients who have pain complaints of the posterior tibial tendon in post-traumatic or post-surgery cases and in patients who have chronic tenosynovitis.

The authors believe that an endoscopic synovectomy in rheumatoid arthritis can preserve the posterior tibial tendon for a period of time and thereby prevent the development of a pes planovalgus. Especially in patients who have rheumatoid arthritis, it is important to avoid immobilization with plaster and mobilization with crutches to prevent (further) damage to other joints.

Summary

Between 1994 and 2004, 33 patients underwent an endoscopic procedure of the posterior tibial tendon. The pathology was diverse. None of the patients showed postoperative complications. All showed a quick recovery, early mobilization, none or mild postoperative pain, and nice wound healing. Although not all patients were free of complaints, all were satisfied with the intervention itself.

References

[1] Myerson M, Solomon G, Shereff M. Posterior tibial tendon dysfunction: its association with seronegative inflammatory disease. Foot Ankle 1989;9:219–25.

[2] Trnka HJ. Dysfunction of the tendon of tibialis posterior. J Bone Joint Surg Br 2004;7: 939–46.

[3] Miller SD, van Holsbeeck M, Boruta PM, et al. Ultrasound in the diagnosis of the diagnosis of the posterior tibial tendon pathology. Foot Ankle Int 1996;17(9):555–8.

[4] Van Dijk CN, Kort N, Scholten P. Tendoscopy of the posterior tibial tendon. Arthoscopy 1997;6:692–8.

[5] Bare AA, Hadded SL. Tenosynovitis of the posterior tibial tendon. Foot Ankle Clin 2001;6: 37–66.

[6] Michelson J, Easley M, Wigley FM, et al. Posterior tibial tendon dysfunction in rheumatoid arthritis. Foot Ankle Int 1995;16(3):156–61.

[7] Paus AC. Arthroscopic synovectomy. When, which diseases and which joints. Z Rheumatol 1996;55:394–400.

[8] Van Dijk CN, Scholten PE, Kort NP. Tendoscopy (tendon sheath endoscopy) for overuse tendon injuries. Oper Tech Sport Med 1997;5(3):170–8.

[9] Van Dijk CN, Kort NP. Tendoscopy of the peroneal tendons. Arthroscopy 1998;14(5):471–8.

[10] Wertheimer SJ, Weber CA, Loder BG, et al. The role of endoscopy in treatment of posterior tibial synovitis. J Foot Ankle Surg 1995;34(1):15–22.

[11] Lapididus PW, Seidenstein H. Chronic non-specific tenosynovitis with effusion about the ankle. J Bone Joint Surg Am 1950;32:175–9.

ELSEVIER
SAUNDERS

Foot Ankle Clin N Am
11 (2006) 429–438

FOOT AND
ANKLE CLINICS

Achilles Tendoscopy

Ferry Steenstra, MD*, C. Niek van Dijk, MD, PhD

*Department of Orthopaedic Surgery, Academic Medical Centre Amsterdam, P.O. Box 22660,
1100 DD, Amsterdam, The Netherlands*

Endoscopic surgery provides easy access to the narrow space around the Achilles tendon and the paratenon. The diagnostic process and the decision for a surgical treatment versus a nonsurgical treatment are the same as for conventional open surgery. Endoscopic surgery offers the advantages that are related to any minimally invasive procedure, such as smaller wounds, fewer wound infections, less blood loss, and less morbidity.

Anatomy

General anatomy

It is possible, even in obese patients, to palpate the medial and lateral borders of the Achilles tendon. Important bony landmarks are the posterior aspect of the calcaneus and the medial and lateral malleolus. The Achilles tendon, or calcaneal tendon, is the strongest and thickest tendon in the human body. It is approximately 12 cm to 15 cm long, and is a fusion of the aponeurosis of the soleus muscle and the gastrocnemius muscle. Typically, the insertion of the Achilles tendon is located 2 cm to 3 cm distal to the superior portion of the posterior process of the calcaneus. In the course of the tendon there is a lateral twist of 90°. The fibers of the gastrocnemius muscle insert at the lateral aspect of the posterior surface of the calcaneus, and the fibers of the soleus muscle insert at the medial aspect of the posterior surface of the calcaneus. The Achilles tendon does not have a tendon sheath but is surrounded by a paratenon. In the space between the ventral side of the distal part of the Achilles tendon—just before its insertion on the calcaneus—is the retrocalcaneal bursa, which can be inflamed.

---

* Corresponding author.
E-mail address: steenstraf@hotmail.com (F. Steenstra).

1083-7515/06/$ – see front matter © 2006 Elsevier Inc. All rights reserved.
doi:10.1016/j.fcl.2006.02.001

The plantaris tendon runs just medial to the distal Achilles tendon. The proximal attachment of the plantaris muscle is the inferior aspect of the lateral supracondylar line of the femur adjacent to its popliteal surface and the posterolateral aspect of the capsule of the knee joint. The long tendon of the plantaris runs in a distal direction, after its small muscle belly, between the medial head of the gastrocnemius muscle and the underlying soleus muscle. Its insertion is on the medial side of the posterior surface of the calcaneus. The plantaris muscle is a weak flexor of the knee and a weak plantar flexor of the ankle. The plantaris tendon is present in most, but not all, patients. The the plantaris tendon, the Achilles tendon, and the paratendineum are extremely close, especially in a combined tendinopathy and paratendinopathy.

Important structures are found just anterior to the Achilles tendon. The tendons of the peroneus longus and brevis are located just behind the lateral malleolus. The flexor muscle hallucis longus runs just anterior to the Achilles tendon. The neural and vascular structures as well as the flexor digitorum longus and posterior tibial tendon are located more medially.

Specific anatomy

A paratenon is located around the Achilles tendon, instead of a real tendon sheath. This paratenon is divided into parietal and visceral layers. The mesotenon connects the outer parietal layer to the inner visceral layer, and is the site for the blood supply. The tendon receives blood of osseous and periosteal vessels at the insertion of the Achilles tendon. There is little blood supply to the distal part of the Achilles tendon. This is one of the reasons why degenerative changes often are located in this area. The limited blood supply often causes a prolonged recovery.

Before the limb is exsanguinated take notice of the short saphenous vein, which runs just laterally, from the lateral border of the Achilles tendon and posterior of the lateral malleolus. The sural nerve runs along with the short saphenous vein, which also should be preserved [1,2].

Etiology

Chronic tendinopathy has a high prevalence in older athletes. Thirty percent of running injuries are caused by overuse [3]. Clement and colleagues theorized that tendon injuries are caused by microtrauma. They are produced by eccentric loading by fatigued muscles or excess tendon loading because of limb position [4].

An inflammatory reaction rarely is found in the tendon. Alfredson and colleagues studied tendons in symptomatic patients using microdialysis, and found no signs of inflammation [5]. They concluded that "tendinitis" is an inaccurate diagnosis. Biopsies of Achilles tendons in symptomatic patients who had overuse injuries showed different histologic findings, including calcifications, fibrocartilaginous metaplasia, hyaline degeneration, fatty degeneration, and myxoid degeneration. These studies were performed on biopsies of tendons that were taken during surgery, not on tendons that were treated conservatively. Rehabilitation programs, often consisting of eccentric exercises, can treat many overuse injuries with a high rate of success [3].

Structure of the Achilles tendon on the cellular level

The Achilles tendon structure is formed by fascicles that are separated by endotenon. The tendon itself is made of tenocytes, a mature type of fibroblasts. These cells are located in a extracellular matrix that is made of elastin, collagen, glycoproteins, and mucopolysaccharides.

Classification of Achilles tendon–related problems

Pathology of the Achilles tendon can be divided into noninsertional or insertional problems [6,7]. The first type can present as local, often cystic degeneration of the Achilles tendon that can be combined with paratendinopathy. Insertional problems are related to abnormalities at the insertion of the Achilles tendon, and include the posterior aspect of the calcaneus and the retrocalcaneal bursa.

Noninsertional Achilles tendon–related problems

Noninsertional pathology can be divided into three entities: tendinopathy, paratendinopathy, and a combination of the two. Symptoms include painful swelling, typically 4 cm to 6 cm proximal to the insertion.

Patients who have tendinopathy can present with three patterns: diffuse thickening of the tendon, local degeneration of the tendon (visualized well on MRI) but it is mechanically intact, or insufficiency of the tendon with a (partial) rupture. In a paratendinopathy there is painful swelling of the paratenon. On MRI, the signal of the Achilles tendon is normal and only the paratenon is involved. Paratendinopathy can be acute or chronic. Often, the pain is more prominent on the medial side in patients who have chronic paratendinopathy [8].

Medially, the soleus tendon and the plantaris tendon are separated from the paratenon. Some investigators suggested that degeneration of the soleus tendon was a possible explanation for this localized, medial pain. Pronation of the foot places greater forces on the medial part of the Achilles tendon.

Degeneration was found during autopsies in 34% of tendons in patients without complaints [9]. Therefore, it is questionable if degeneration in the tendon itself is the main cause of the pain. The authors believe that it is more likely that the accompanying paratendinopathy gives rise to the symptoms.

The plantaris tendon is located on the medial side. In contrast to the adjacent soleus muscle the plantaris muscle is biarticular, because it inserts from the distal femur, whereas the soleus muscle inserts onto the tibia. Simultaneous knee and ankle movements result in a different pull of both tendons at the level of the combined tendinopathy and paratendinopathy. In a healthy patient the plantaris tendon can glide in relation to the Achilles tendon. Because of the chronic paratendinopathy the plantaris tendon is more or less fixed to the Achilles tendon at the level of the nodule. Distal pull by means of repetitive hyperpronation or proximal pull by means of the separate biarticular muscle belly of the plantaris tendon may provide an explanation for this medial pain.

Overuse is an important factor that contributes to this entity. Other factors that were described in literature include malalignment, errors in training, strength imbalance, compression and friction of the tendon, shoe-related complaints, inactivity, rheumatoid arthritis (RA), endocrine disorders, and drugs.

Diagnoses to be excluded are peroneal tendinopathy; tendinitis of the tibialis posterior tendon; tendinitis of the flexor hallucis longus; posterior subtalar arthritis; posterior ankle impingement; ankle arthritis; tarsal tunnel syndrome; seronegative arthritis (spondylitis, reactive arthritis); and systemic diseases, including seropositive arthritis (RA, lupus) [3].

Operative treatment of tendinopathy depends on the stage of the disease. Local degeneration and thickening usually are treated by excision and curettage. An insufficient Achilles tendon that is due to gross degeneration is treated by reconstruction. Isolated paratendinopathy usually is treated by excision. Debridement of the Achilles tendon, combined with a decompression of the fascia (fasciotomy), was advised by Quist and Quist.

In combined tendinopathy and paratendinopathy, the question is whether both pathologies need to be treated. Because it is questionable whether the local tendinopathy contributes to the clinical presentation [9], the authors focus on treatment of the paratendinopathy. Their current approach is an endoscopic release of the plantar tendon at the level of the nodule and removal of the local paratendinopathy.

Alfredson and colleagues [10] described neovascularization around the Achilles tendon as a possible cause of pain at the level of a tendinopathy nodule. In a patient who has combined tendinopathy and paratendinopathy and a proven neovascularization on ultrasound, a microdialysis using polidocanol can be performed [11].

Diagnosis

Physical examination

The Achilles tendon can be palpated easily. Swelling and local tenderness are detected. Differentiation between a tendinopathy and a paratendinopathy is important. In the case of an insertional tendinopathy, the pain on palpation usually is located in the midportion of the insertion at the calcaneus. In the case of a retrocalcaneal bursitis, the thickened bursa can be palpated just medially and laterally from the Achilles tendon and directly proximal to the dorsal aspect of the calcaneus.

In the case of tendinopathy, a tender nodular swelling—typically 4 cm to 6 cm proximal to the insertion onto the calcaneus—moves up and down during passive plantarflexion and dorsiflexion. When there is a paratendinopathy this swelling does not move during passive plantarflexion and dorsiflexion.

Radiology

Kager's triangle, the fat pad just anterior to the Achilles tendon, can be detected on a plain lateral radiograph. The triangle is disturbed in chronic inflammation. In cases of retrocalcaneal bursitis the lateral radiograph shows a disturbance of Kager's triangle. Because of infiltration of water into the fat pad there are more gray and less black colors in the triangle.

A good image of the Achilles tendon can be given by ultrasound. The level of experience of the radiologist is important. The retrocalcaneal bursa and a local nodule can be identified with ultrasound. Ultrasound can be used in combination with a Doppler flow measurement to judge if neovascularization is present. MRI can be performed in cases of chronic tendinopathy.

Achilles tendon pathology can be classified as tendinopathy, paratendinopathy, or a combination. In Achilles tendinopathy there are intrinsic or intrasubstance inflammatory changes of the Achilles tendon. In paratendinopathy there is inflammation of the paratenon. An irregular pre-Achilles fat pad may be seen with paratendinopathy. MRI findings in Achilles tendinopathy include fusiform thickening of the Achilles tendon and diffuse or linear low to intermediate signal intensity on T2-weighted, fat-suppressed; T2-weighted fast spin-echo; or STIR images. Fat-suppressed and T2-weighted fast spin-echo sequences are not as sensitive to intrasubstance signal intensity as are T2-weighted or STIR techniques. Sagittal MRIs can demonstrate an anterior convexity or a local enlargement of the Achilles tendon. In cases of retrocalcaneal bursitis, the sagittal images show an extension of fluid in the retrocalcaneal bursa. It can be difficult to distinguish areas of tendinopathy from intrasubstance tendon tears. Adhesion between the paratenon and the Achilles tendon is associated with paratendinopathy.

The MRI of a local Achilles tendon tear shows local thickening without an increased signal intensity [12].

Differential diagnosis

Pathology of the tendons of the peroneus longus and brevis, intra-articular pathology of the ankle joint and subtalar joint, degenerative changes of the posterior tibial tendon, and tendinitis of the flexor muscle hallucis longus must be ruled out.

Treatment

Conservative treatment is the treatment of choice. Modification of the activity level of the patient is advised together with avoidance of strenuous activities in cases of paratendinopathy. Shoe modifications and inlays are given. Physical therapy includes stretching and icing. Application of a short leg cast can be a next step. Because of the absence of inflammation, the rationale for using nonsteroidal anti-inflammatory drugs is unclear; however, they can play a role in the reduction of pain. The use of oral or injectable steroids is controversial. Degeneration and an increased risk for a subsequent rupture can be promoted by injections around or in the Achilles tendon.

Because the outcome is not always predictable, results of surgical treatment of Achilles tendinopathy can be frustrating for the patient and the surgeons [13]. Decompression of the tendon by incision and excision of degenerative tissue is performed in an open surgical treatment of an Achilles tendinopathy. The thickened paratenon is excised in cases of paratendinopathy.

This article describes the minimally invasive treatment of chronic combined paratendinopathy and tendinopathy, and the endoscopic treatment of retrocalcaneal bursitis (Haglund's syndrome).

Operative techniques

Anesthesia and patient position

Local, epidural, spinal, or general anesthesia can be used during the procedure in an outpatient surgery setting. The patient is in a prone position. A tourniquet is placed around the upper thigh. The affected foot is placed at the end of the table because the surgeon must be able to move the foot in full dorsiflexion and plantarflexion.

Arthroscopic instruments

The small-diameter short arthroscope yields an excellent picture that is difficult to distinguish from that obtained with a standard 4-mm arthroscope; therefore, a 2.7-mm arthroscope with 30° obliquity can be used. The small diameter arthroscope sheath, however, cannot deliver the same amount of irrigation fluid per time as can the standard 4-mm sheath. This is important in procedures in which a large-diameter shaver is used (eg, reduction of Haglund's syndrome). The authors use a 2.7-mm arthroscope for endoscopic treatment of a combined tendinopathy and paratendinopathy [4].

Irrigation

Different fluids, including Ringer's lactate, normal saline, or glycine, can be used for arthroscopic irrigation. When a 4-mm arthroscope is used, gravity inflow usually is sufficient. A pressurized bag or pump device sometimes is used with the 2.7-mm arthroscope [4].

Other instruments

In addition to the standard endoscopic equipment a probe and an endoscopic shaver system are used.

Operative technique of noninsertional pathology of the Achilles tendon

General principles

The patient is in a prone position with both feet positioned at the end of the table. Epidural, spinal, or general anesthesia can be used. The short saphenous vein is marked on the lateral side of the Achilles tendon before inflating the tourniquet, which is positioned around the upper leg.

Portals

The distal portal is located on the lateral border of the Achilles tendon 2 cm to 3 cm distal to the pathologic thickened nodule. The cranial portal is located 2 cm to 4 cm above the nodule on the medial border of the Achilles tendon. Thus, it usually is possible to visualize and work around the whole surface of the tendon over a length of approximately 10 cm. The distal portal is made first. After making the skin incision, a mosquito clamp is introduced which is followed by the blunt 2.7-mm trocar in a craniolateral direction. In the same direction—looking ventrally over the edge of the tendon on the craniolateral side—the 2.7-mm arthroscope with an inclination angle of 30° is introduced. Identification of the Achilles tendon is easy at the level of a healthy part of the tendon. To minimize the risk of iatrogenic damage to neurovascular structures keep the arthroscope on the tendon. The proximal portal is made in the same manner by introducing a spinal needle, followed by a mosquito clamp and probe. The plantaris tendon is now identified just medial to the Achilles tendon. In a typical case of local paratendinopathy the plantar tendon, the Achilles tendon, and the paratendineum are tight together in the inflammatory process (Fig. 1). Removal of the local thickened inflamed paratendineum and release of the plantaris tendon are the goals of this procedure (Figs. 2 and 3).

A resection of the paratenon is performed on the anterior side of the tendon at the level of the painful nodule. The neovascularization, which is accompanied by small nerve fibers, can be found in this area. These neurovascular endings can

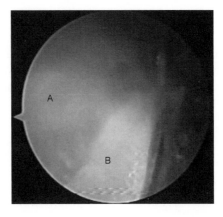

Fig. 1. Intraoperative photograph of an a noninsertional paratendinopathy of the Achilles tendon. This shows the close relationship between the Achilles tendon (*A*) and the plantaris tendon (*B*) before the release is performed.

be removed by blunt dissection with the trocar followed by removal of tissue with the full-radius 2.7-mm resector shaver.

Changing portals can be helpful. At the end of the procedure it must be possible to move the arthroscope over the complete symptomatic area of the Achilles tendon.

Intraoperative complications

Equipment breakage

Although equipment has improved, breakage can occur in less than 0.1% of cases [14]. Removal of broken pieces can be difficult and can cause tissue damage.

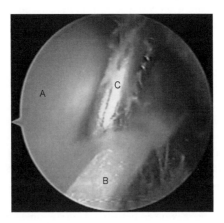

Fig. 2. Intraoperative photograph of the same patient as in Fig. 1. The clamp (*C*) is between the Achilles tendon (*A*) and the plantaris tendon (*B*) to perform the release.

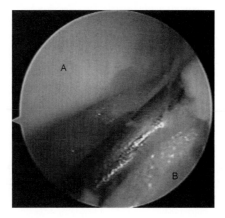

Fig. 3. Intraoperative photograph of the same patient as Figs. 1 and 2. The release has been performed. There is space between the Achilles tendon (*A*) and the plantaris tendon (*B*).

Vascular injuries and nerve lesions

Neural and vascular injuries are rare; however, the neurovascular structures can be close to the surgical field on the medial side.

Postoperative complications

Wound healing problems can occur, and are described in 30% of patients after an open surgical procedure for an Achilles tendon problem [8]. Wound healing problems after endoscopic surgery are almost nonexistent [15,16].

Aftercare

The patient is allowed full weight bearing if tolerated. The compressive dressing is applied for 2 or 3 days. Initially, the foot must be elevated when not walking. An active range of motion of the ankle is encouraged [15].

Outcome

The authors treated 20 successive patients with an endoscopic release for a noninsertional tendinopathy combined with a paratendinopathy. All patients had had complaints for more than 2 years. The results were analyzed with a follow-up of 2–7 years with a mean of 6 years. Sixteen patients were seen for follow-up, which included a Foot and Ankle Outcome Score (FAOS) questionnaire and a short-form health survey with only 36 questions (SF-36).

There were no complications. Most patients were able to resume their sporting activities after 4 to 8 weeks. All patients had significant pain relief. The FAOS and SF-36 score were comparable to a cohort of people without Achilles tendon complaints.

One comparable study by Maquirrain and colleagues [16] reported on seven patients who underwent an endoscopic release for chronic Achilles tendino-pathies. Their results were similar. The mean score (on a scale of 100) of this group improved from 39 preoperatively to 89 postoperatively, and there were no complications.

Summary

Endoscopic release for a noninsertional tendinopathy combined with a para-tendinopathy gives good clinical results, and has the advantages that are related to any minimally invasive procedure.

References

[1] Hamilton WG. Surgical anatomy of the foot and ankle. Clin Symp 1985;37(3):2–32.
[2] Hoppenfeld S, de Boer P. Surgical exposures in orthopaedics: the anatomic approach. Phila-delphia: Lippincott Co.; 1994.
[3] Lysholm J, Wiklander J. Injuries in runners. Am J Sports Med 1987;15(2):168–71.
[4] van Dijk CN. Ankle joint arthroscopy. In: DuParc J, editor. Surgical techniques in orthopaedics and traumatology, vol. 8. Paris: Elsevier; 2003.
[5] Fitzgerald RH, Kaufer H, Malkani AL. Overuse injuries. In: Kaufer H, editor. Othopaedics. 1st edition. St. Louis (MO): Mosby; 2002. p. 554–6.
[6] Saltzman C, Bonar S. Tendon problems of the foot and ankle. In: Lutter LD, Mizel MS, Pfeffer GB, editors. Orthopaedic knowledge update –foot and ankle. Rosemont (IL): American Acad-emy of Orthopaedic Surgeons; 1994. p. 269–82.
[7] Clain MR, Baxter DE. Achilles tendinitis. Foot Ankle 1992;13:482–7.
[8] Segesser B, Goesele A, Rengli P. The Achilles tendon in sports. Orthopade 1995;24(3):252–67.
[9] Kannus P, et al. Histopathological changes preceding spontaneous rupture of a tendon. J Bone Joint Surg 1991;73A(10):1507–25.
[10] Alfredson H, Thorsen K, Lorentson R, et al. In situ microdialysis in tendon tissue: high levels of glutamate but not prostaglandin E2 in chronic Achilles tendon pain. Knee Surg Sports Traumatol Arthrosc 1999;7:378–81.
[11] Alfredson H, Ohberg L. Sclerosing injections to areas of neo-vascularisation reduce pain in chronic Achilles tendinopathy: a double-blind randomised controlled trial. Knee Surg Sports Traumatol Arthrosc 2005;13(4):338–44.
[12] Ko R, Porter M. Interactive foot and ankle 2. London: Primal Pictures; 2000.
[13] Maffulli N, Binfield PM, Moore D, et al. Surgical decompression of chronic central core lesions of the Achilles tendon. Am J Sports Med 1999;27(6):747–52.
[14] Sprague NF. Complications in arthroscopic surgery. New York: Raven Press; 1989.
[15] van Dijk CN, van Dyk GE, Scholten PE, et al. Endoscopic calcaneoplasty. Am J Sports Med 2001;29(2):185–9.
[16] Maquirrain J, et al. Endoscopic surgery in chronic Achilles tendinopathies : a preliminary report. Arthroscopy 2002;18(3):298–303.

ELSEVIER
SAUNDERS

Foot Ankle Clin N Am
11 (2006) 439–446

FOOT AND
ANKLE CLINICS

Endoscopic Calcaneoplasty

Peter E. Scholten, MD[a],*, C. Niek van Dijk, MD, PhD[b]

[a]*Department of Orthopaedic Surgery, "Kliniek Klein Rosendael," Rosendaalselaan 30, 6891 DG Rozendaal, The Netherlands*
[b]*Department of Orthopaedic Surgery, Academic Medical Center, P.O. Box 22660, 1100 DD Amsterdam, The Netherlands*

Pain on the posterior aspect of the heel can be a disabling condition. When the pain is caused by a complex of symptoms of a posterosuperior calcaneal prominence and retrocalcaneal bursitis, it is called Haglund's syndrome. Originally, Haglund [1] described a painful hindfoot that was caused by an enlarged posterosuperior calcaneal border in combination with the wearing of rigid low-back shoes. Today, Haglund's disease is characterized by pain and tenderness at the posterolateral aspect of the calcaneus where a calcaneal prominence can be palpated. This entity also is known as "pump-bump." A distinction between Haglund's disease and other pathologic conditions, such as a superficial Achilles bursitis, must be made. Haglund's syndrome involves a painful swelling of an inflamed retrocalcaneal bursa, sometimes combined with insertional tendinopathy of the Achilles tendon. The syndrome is caused by repetitive impingement of the bursa between the ventral aspect of the Achilles tendon and the posterosuperior calcaneal prominence. Typically, patients have pain when they start to walk after a period of rest. Operative treatment consists of removal of the inflamed bursa and resection of the bony prominence. A distinction should be made with other pathologies in this region.

Achilles tendon pathology can be divided into insertional and noninsertional problems [2,3]. Noninsertional pathology can be divided into tendinopathy, paratendinopathy, or a combination of these two. Symptoms typically occur 4 cm to 6 cm above the insertion. Tendinopathy at the insertion is called insertional tendinopathy. Often, the pain is located in the midline at the insertion onto the calcaneus. Insertional tendinopathy can exist in combination with a retrocalcaneal

---

* Corresponding author.
E-mail address: pscholten@medinova.com (P.E. Scholten).

bursitis. In retrocalcaneal bursitis, as part of Haglund's syndrome, pain can be reproduced by palpation laterally and medially of the Achilles tendon at the level of the posterosuperior border of the calcaneus. Pain is elicited with dorsiflexion of the ankle because impingement of the retrocalcaneal bursa occurs between the anterior border of the Achilles tendon and the posterior superior rim of the calcaneus, which leads to retrocalcaneal bursitis (Fig. 1).

Conservative treatment for retrocalcaneal bursitis includes avoidance of tight shoes, adaptation of activities, nonsteroidal anti-inflammatory drugs (NSAIDs), the use of padding, physical therapy, and a single injection of corticosteroids into the retrocalcaneal space. Two surgical methods prevail when conservative treatment fails. Operative techniques mainly consists of an open resection of the posterior superior part of the calcaneus or a calcaneal wedge osteotomy. Complications of the open surgical treatment can be superficial or deep. Skin breakdown, tenderness around the operative scar, unsightly operative scars, or altered sensation around the heel can occur [4–8]. Other complications, such as Achilles tendon avulsion, weakening of the osseous structure when an enlargement of the entire posterosuperior aspect of the calcaneus is removed, and calcaneal stress fractures, have been described [4,7,9]. Recurrent pain secondary to an inadequate amount of bone resected, and stiffness of the Achilles tendon that results in

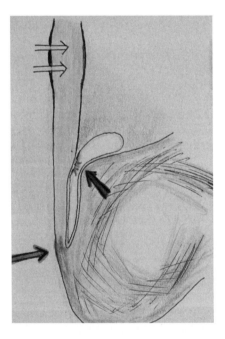

Fig. 1. Red arrow points to the retrocalcaneal bursa being impinged by the superoposterior edge of the calcaneus and the Achilles tendon. White and green arrows indicate the typical locations of noninsertional and insertional tendinopathy, respectively, of the Achilles tendon.

decreased dorsiflexion also have been reported [10]. Wound healing problems after open surgery have been described in 30% of patients [11]. Endoscopic treatment offers the advantages that are related to any minimally invasive procedure, such as low morbidity, excellent scar healing, functional aftertreatment, short recovery time, and quick sports resumption. In 2001 the authors published their initial results, which was a combined series of patients that was treated in our hospital, and patients that were treated by van Dyk who used a slightly different technique (patient in the supine position) [12]. This article describes the technique and results and the results of a consecutive group of patients that was treated in the prone position in the authors' hospital.

Surgical technique

The operation is performed under general or regional anesthesia with the patient in a prone position. An Esmarch bandage is used to exsanguinate the leg, and a thigh tourniquet is inflated. The feet are positioned just at the edge of the operating table. The involved leg is elevated slightly by placing a small support under the lower leg. The foot is plantarflexed by gravity. Dorsiflexion of the foot can be controlled by pressure from the surgeon's body against the plantarflexed foot, which keeps both hands free to manipulate the arthroscope and instruments. The lateral portal is made first. A small vertical incision is made through the skin at the level of the superior aspect of the calcaneus. The retrocalcaneal space is penetrated by a blunt trocar. A 4.5-mm arthroscope shaft with an inclination angle of 30° is introduced. A 70° arthroscope also can be useful, but seldom is necessary (Fig. 2). Under direct vision a spinal needle is introduced just medial to the Achilles tendon, again at the level of the superior aspect of the calcaneus, to locate the medial portal. After making a vertical stab incision, the 5.0-mm full-radius resector is placed and visualized by the arthroscope. The inflamed retrocalcaneal bursa is removed to provide a better view. The superior surface of the calcaneus is visualized, and its fibrous layer and periosteum is stripped off. All of the time the opening of the shaver is facing the bone. When the foot is brought into full dorsiflexion, the impingement site is determined. The foot is placed in full plantarflexion and the posterior superior bone rim can be removed (Fig. 3). This bone is soft and is removed easily by the aggressive synovial full-radius resector/bone cutter. A burr is not needed at this point. The two portals can be used interchangeably for the arthroscope and the resector to remove all of the bony prominence. It is important to remove enough bone at the posteromedial and lateral corner. These edges have to be rounded off by moving the synovial resector beyond the posterior edge onto the lateral medial wall of the calcaneus. The Achilles tendon is protected throughout the procedure by keeping the closed end of the resector against the tendon. The insertion of the Achilles tendon can be found with the foot in the fully plantarflexed position. The synovial resector is placed on the insertion against the calcaneus to smooth this part of the calcaneus. During this part of the procedure, fluoroscopic verification of the position of the

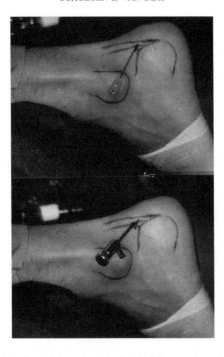

Fig. 2. A lateral portal is made at the level of the superior calcaneal rim.

synovial resector can be helpful. A burr or small acromionizer can be introduced for removing the hard cortical bone at the attachment of the Achilles tendon. Switching portals should be done to ensure that sufficient medial and lateral bone is removed. Finally, the resector is placed to clean up loose debris and to smooth rough edges. To prevent sinus formation, the skin incisions are sutured and a

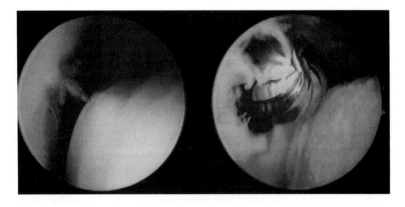

Fig. 3. Resection of the superoposterior calcaneal rim with a burr.

compressive dressing is applied. Postoperatively, the patient is allowed weight bearing as tolerated, and is instructed to elevate the foot when not walking. The dressing is removed 3 days postoperatively, and the patient is allowed to shower. The patient is encouraged to do active range of motion exercises for at least 10 minutes three times a day. The patient is allowed to return to regular shoewear as soon as it is tolerated.

Patients

Between 1995 and 2000 39 procedures were performed in 36 patients: 20 men and 16 women. The average age was 35.0 years (range, 16–50 years). Eighteen procedures were performed on the left side and 21 were performed on the right side. A systematic history was taken in all patients that included etiology, pain (at rest, and when standing, walking, running, walking uphill, and walking on a hard surface), duration of complaints, physical requirements at work, and level of sports participation. The physical examination included the assessment of leg length discrepancy; lower extremity axis; gait disturbance; range of motion of ankle, subtalar joint and foot; local swelling and warmth; pain on palpation; location of the pain on palpation; and pain on Achilles tendon stretch.

The patients had a painful swelling of the soft tissues of the posterior heel, medial and lateral to the Achilles tendon. Stretching the Achilles tendon was painful, without pain on palpation of the tendon itself. Two patients had a mild cavovarus deformity. Radiographs were taken routinely. Initially, all cases had a superior calcaneal angle of more than 75° and all patients had positive parallel pitch lines. Because the authors' initial results were good [12], the indication was expanded to include patients who did not meet the radiographic criteria. Some patients presented the identical clinical picture, but had a less pronounced superior calcaneal angle. All patients were refractory to conservative treatment for at least 6 months. Conservative treatment, including rest, physical therapy, NSAIDs, and heel support did not alleviate the pain. Four patients had a period of plaster immobilization. Four patients had failure of open surgery and recurrence of the deformity. The mean follow-up was 4.5 years (range, 2–7.5 years). There were no surgical complications, except for 1 patient who experienced a small area of hypoesthesia over the heel pad. There were no postoperative infections or sore or unsightly scars. All patients were pleased with their small incisions. Only 2 patients were not improved. Four patients had fair results, 6 patients had good results, and 24 patients had excellent results (Ogilvie-Harris score). Patients who considered their results to be fair had residual complaints; two of them had a cavovarus deformity. The average recovery period was 8 weeks for the groups that had good and excellent results [4–16]. Work resumption took place at an average of 5 weeks (range, 10 days–6 months). Sports resumption took place at an average of 11 weeks (range, 6 weeks–6 months). Some swelling usually was present up to 3 months after surgery. One patient had a delayed healing of one of the incisions (2 weeks).

Discussion

Conservative therapy for retrocalcaneal bursitis includes a single, diagnostic infiltration in the retrocalcaneal bursa with corticosteroids [10,13,14] after other treatments have failed. There is a potential for rupture of the Achilles tendon with repeated injections; therefore, this is not advised. The operative treatment of retrocalcaneal bursitis after failure of conservative measures aims at prevention of impingement of the retrocalcaneal bursa between the Achilles tendon and the os calcis. This can be accomplished by removal of the inflamed retrocalcaneal bursa followed by resection of the superoposterior calcaneal prominence or a dorsal closing-wedge osteotomy.

Superoposterior calcaneal resection can be performed by way of a posterolateral incision, a posteromedial incision, or both [5,8,15]. Endoscopic calcaneoplasty offers a good alternative to open resection. Surgeons who are accustomed to the arthroscope will find the endoscopic approach more rewarding than an open procedure because of better visualization. Poor results after open partial calcaneal resection for retrocalcaneal bursitis have been reported [5,16]. The time to sports resumption after this resection can be up to 9 months [10]. The authors' patient series shows a high percentage of good and excellent results. Advantages of the endoscopic technique are that complications, such as wound dehiscence, painful or unsightly scars, and nerve entrapment within the scar, can be avoided. Inappropriate tendon visualization during open surgery can weaken the Achilles tendon insertion and can cause tendon rupture [7,9]. Disagreement exists regarding the appropriate surgical approach (ie, medial, lateral, or both) [5,8,17].

Jones and James [17] performed 10 partial dorsal calcaneal ostectomies for retrocalcaneal bursitis; aftertreatment consisted of 8 weeks in a short leg walking cast followed by a rehabilitation program. All patients had reached their desired activity level within 6 months. Angermann [5] operated on 40 heels in 37 patients for the same indication using a posterolateral incision and allowed immediate weight bearing. Complications included one case of superficial heel infection, one case of hematoma, and two cases of delayed skin healing. At an average follow-up of 6 years, 50% of the patients were cured, 20% were improved, 20% were unchanged, and 10% were worse. In a study by Pauker and colleagues [8], 28 heels were operated on in 22 patients who had retrocalcaneal bursitis. All wore a short leg walking cast for 4 weeks. At follow-up (mean 13 years), 15 of 19 patients had a good result. The investigators advocated using one incision, because many patients have complaints of tenderness over the operative scar for up to 1 year after surgery which might be exaggerated by an extensive approach. In a study by Schepsis and colleagues [16] of 24 patients who had retrocalcaneal bursitis, 6 (25%) patients had a fair result that required reoperation. Huber and Waldis [6] found a considerable amount of residual complaints in 32 patients who were examined clinically and radiologically at a mean follow-up of 18.6 years after being treated for Haglund's exostoses by resection of the posterosuperior calcaneal prominence. Fourteen of the 32 patients had soft tissue problems, including excessive scar formation and persistent swelling. Not enough bone was removed in 8 patients and 2 patients had new bone formation; both caused persistent painful swelling. In 8 patients a disturbance in Achilles tendon function was noted. The open operative treatment of retrocalcaneal bursitis requires good exposure to remove an adequate amount of bone. Conversely, a large exposure is accompanied by a significant percentage of wound and soft tissue problems.

Arthroscopic surgery allows for excellent medial and lateral visualization. Thus, the Achilles tendon and its insertion and the calcaneus can be inspected and treated. This minimizes the chance of removing and disturbing the Achilles tendon attachment. Some surgeons who use the open technique [17–19] advise postoperative plaster immobilization, which carries the risk for new adhesions and scar tissue formation. The endoscopic treatment has the advantage of functional aftertreatment; thereby, late complications, such as stiffness and pain, are avoided. Jerosch and Nasef [20] used the same technique and published the same good results.

Summary

Whether the operation is performed by endoscopic or open technique, enough bone has to be removed to prevent impingement of the retrocalcaneal bursa between the calcaneus and Achilles tendon. The endoscopic calcaneoplasty has several advantages, including low morbidity, functional aftertreatment, outpatient treatment, excellent scar healing, a short recovery time, and quick sports resumption, in comparison with the open technique.

References

[1] Haglund P. Beitrag zur Klinik der Achillessehne [Article on clinical pathology of the Achilles tendon]. Zeitschr Orthop Chir 1928;49:49–58 [in German].

[2] Clain MR, Baxter DE. Achilles tendinitis. Foot Ankle 1992;13(8):482–7.

[3] Saltzman CL, Tearse DS. Achilles tendon injuries. J Am Acad Orthop Surg 1998;6(5):316–25.

[4] Leach RE, DiIorio E, Harney RA. Pathologic hindfoot conditions in the athlete. Clin Orthop Rel Res 1983;177:116–21.

[5] Angermann P. Chronic retrocalcaneal bursitis treated by resection of the calcaneus. Foot Ankle 1990;10(5):285–7.

[6] Huber HM, Waldis M. Die Haglund-Exostose—eine Operationsindikation und ein kleiner Eingriff? [Haglund's Exostosis—a surgical indication and a minor intervention?]. Z Orthop 1989; 127:286–90 [in German].

[7] Miller AE, Vogel TA. Haglund's deformity and the Keck and Kelly osteotomy: a retrospective analysis. J Foot Surg 1989;28(1):23–9.

[8] Pauker M, Katz K, Yosipovitch Z. Calcaneal ostectomy for Haglund disease. J Foot Surg 1992; 31(6):588–9.

[9] Le TA, Joseph PM. Common exostectomies of the rearfoot. Clin Podiatr Med Surg 1991; 8(3):611–7.

[10] Nesse E, Finsen V. Poor results after resection for Haglund's heel. Analysis of 35 heels in 23 patients after 3 years. Acta Orthop Scand 1994;65(1):107–9.

[11] Segesser B, Goesele A, Renggli P. [The Achilles tendon in sports]. Orthopade 1995;24(3): 252–67.

[12] van Dijk CN, van Dyk GE, Scholten PE, et al. Endoscopic calcaneoplasty. Am J Sports Med 2001;29(2):185–9.

[13] Myerson MS, McGarvey W. Disorders of the insertion of the Achilles tendon and Achilles tendinitis. An instructional course lecture. J Bone Joint Surg 1998;80A(12):1814–24.

[14] Subotnick SI, Block AJ. Retrocalcaneal problems. Clin Podiatr Med Surg 1990;7(2):323–32.

[15] Kolodziej P, Glisson RR, Nunley JA. Risk of avulsion of the Achilles tendon after partial excision for treatment of insertional tendonitis and Haglund's deformity: a biomechanical study. Foot Ankle Int 1999;20(7):433–7.

[16] Schepsis AA, Wagner C, Leach RE. Surgical management of Achilles tendon overuse injuries. A long-term follow-up study. Am J Sports Med 1994;22(5):611–9.

[17] Jones DC, James SL. Partial calcaneal ostectomy for retrocalcaneal bursitis. Am J Sports Med 1984;12(1):72–3.

[18] Hanft JR, Chang T, Levy AI, et al. Grand rounds: Haglund's deformity and retrocalcaneal intratendinous spurring. J Foot Ankle Surg 1996;35(4):362–8.

[19] Paavola M, Orava S, Leppilahti J, et al. Chronic achilles tendon overuse injury: complications after surgical management. An analysis of 432 consecutive patients. Am J Sports Med 2000; 28(1):77–82.

[20] Jerosch J, Nasef NM. Endoscopic calcaneoplasty–rationale, surgical technique, and early results: a preliminary report. Knee Surg Sports Traumatol Arthrosc 2003;11(3):190–5.

**ELSEVIER
SAUNDERS**

Foot Ankle Clin N Am
11 (2006) 447–450

**FOOT AND
ANKLE CLINICS**

Index

Note: Page numbers of article titles are in **boldface** type.

Moving?

Make sure your subscription moves with you!

To notify us of your new address, find your **Clinics Account Number** (located on your mailing label above your name), and contact customer service at:

E-mail: elspcs@elsevier.com

800-654-2452 (subscribers in the U.S. & Canada)
407-345-4000 (subscribers outside of the U.S. & Canada)

Fax number: 407-363-9661

Elsevier Periodicals Customer Service
6277 Sea Harbor Drive
Orlando, FL 32887-4800

*To ensure uninterrupted delivery of your subscription, please notify us at least 4 weeks in advance of move.